FAST

AND FLAVORFUL

Great Diabetes Meals from Market to Table

by Linda Gassenheimer

 American Diabetes Association.

Director, Book Publishing, Abe Ogden; *Acquisitions Editor*, Victor Van Beuren; *Editor*, Greg Guthrie; *Production Manager*, Melissa Sprott; *Composition*, ADA; *Indexer*, Courtney Rutledge; *Cover Design*, Vis-à-Vis Creative Concepts, Inc.; *Photographer*, Taran Z; *Printer*, QuadGraphics.

Cover photo: Pistachio-Crusted Beef and Vegetable Kabobs, p. 218.

Printed in the United States of America
1 3 5 7 9 10 8 6 4 2

♾ The paper in this publication meets the requirements of the ANSI Standard Z39.48-1992 (permanence of paper).

ADA titles may be purchased for business or promotional use or for special sales. To purchase more than 50 copies of this book at a discount, or for custom editions of this book with your logo, contact the American Diabetes Association at the address below, at booksales@diabetes.org, or by calling 703-299-2046.

American Diabetes Association
1701 North Beauregard Street
Alexandria, Virginia 22311

DOI: 10.2337/9781580404440

Library of Congress Cataloging-in-Publication Data
Gassenheimer, Linda.
 Fast and flavorful : great diabetes meals from market to table / by Linda Gassenheimer.
 p. cm.
 Includes bibliographical references and index.
 ISBN 978-1-58040-444-0 (alk. paper)
 1. Diabetes--Diet therapy--Recipes. I. Title.
 RC662.G365 2011
 641.5'6314--dc23
      2011022590

To my husband, Harold,
for his love,
constant enthusiasm for my work,
and support.

CONTENTS

Acknowledgments   ix
Introduction   1
Shop Smart!   3
Cooking Staples   5

SEAFOOD   7

Balsamic Grilled Tuna and Arugula Pasta

Texas Tuna Burger and Jalapeño Coleslaw

Hot Glazed Tuna Steak with Pecan Spinach Salad

Salmon, Quinoa, and Corn Salad

Chilled Cucumber and Salmon Soup

Poached Salmon with Chive Sauce and Vegetable Fettuccini

Salmon Gazpacho

Whiskey-Soused Salmon with Broccoli and Potatoes

Honey-Soy Glazed Salmon with Asparagus Rice

Almond-Crusted Trout with Penne and Sugar Snap Peas

Cumin-Crusted Snapper with Arroz con Jitomate (Rice with Tomato)

Sicilian Swordfish with Broccoli Linguine

Parmesan Sole with Dilled Potatoes

Fish in a Pouch with Garlic Couscous

Ginger-Teriyaki Steamed Fish and Chinese Noodles

Cajun-Bronzed Mahi-Mahi with Rice and Spinach Pilaf

Halibut in Cider with Saffron Rice

Five-Spice Fillet with Chinese Noodles and Sprouts

Southwestern Fish Fillet with Chipotle Corn and Zucchini

Pecan-Crusted Tilapia with Hot Pepper Succotash

Fish Chowder with Green Salad

Mexican Orange Fillet with Fried Corn and Green Pepper

Sautéed Fish with Pineapple Salsa and Poblano Rice

Braised Chinese Shrimp

Sweet and Sour Shrimp with Brown Rice

Spaghetti del Pescatore (Fisherman's Spaghetti) with Celery and Fennel Salad

Lemon-Pepper Shrimp and Couscous on a Bed of Spinach

Shrimp and Poblano Pepper Tacos with Pinto Bean Salad

Black Bean Soup with Shrimp

Shrimp Mushroom Quesadillas and Black Bean and Tomato Salad

Jerk Shrimp with Rice and Peas

Spicy Shrimp and Peach Salad with Lentils Vinaigrette

Hot Pepper Shrimp with Pimento Endive Salad

Shrimp Caesar Salad

Pan-Seared Scallops and Vegetable Medley Rice

Curry-Kissed Scallops with Carrots and Rice

Pesto Scallops with Fresh Fettuccini

Crab Scampi and Spaghetti

Spaghetti with Clams and Herb Sauce and Italian Salad

Aga Khan's Chicken Curry and Rice

Almond-Grape Chicken Salad with Crunchy Coleslaw

Basque Chicken with Saffron Rice

Black Bean Chicken Chili and Iceberg Salad

Chili Chicken with Southwestern Barley Salad

Chicken Pizzaioli with Fennel and Bean Salad

Chicken Tostadas and Cilantro Tomatoes

Chicken and Garlic Greens with Spicy Sautéed Potatoes

Chicken and Shiitake Yakitori

Chicken and Walnuts in Lettuce Puffs with Chinese Rice

Chinese Salad with Asian Dressing

Coq au Vin (Chicken Stewed in Red Wine) with Brown Rice

Country Mushroom and Sausage Soup with Onion-Garlic Crostini

Crispy Chicken with Ratatouille (Sautéed Provençal Vegetables)

Curried Chicken Pot Pie

Dijon Chicken with Vegetable Quinoa

Grilled Chicken Wraps and Parmesan Corn

Hawaiian Chicken with Pineapple Salad

Honey-Spiced Mock Chicken Wings and Celery with Blue Cheese Dressing

Indian-Spiced Chicken with Cumin-Scented Rice and Spinach

Chicken Diavolo (Italian Chicken in Spicy Tomato Sauce) with Zucchini Carrot Gratinée

Jacques Pepin's Supreme of Chicken with Balsamic Vinegar and Onion Sauce with Corn and Peas

Marsala-Glazed Chicken with Roman Spinach

Mexican Sope (Layered Open Tortilla Sandwich)

Pistachio-Crusted Chicken and Broccoli Farfalle

Poached Chicken with Fresh Tomato Mayonnaise Sauce and Cucumber Rice Salad

Pollo Tonnato (Chicken in Tuna Sauce)

Sherry Chicken and Green Bean Pimento Rice

Tarragon Chicken with Orzo and Chives

Thai Chicken Kabobs with Brown Rice

Turkey and Apple Salad with Herbed Cheese Crostini

Turkey Normandy with Sweet Potatoes

Turkey Picadillo with Brown Rice

Turkey Stroganoff with Egg Noodles

Balsamic Pork Scaloppini with Garlic Sweet Potatoes and Sugar Snap Peas

Beer-Soused Pork with Potato and Leeks

Brandied Apples and Pork with Egg Noodles

Chimichurri Pork Chops with Quick Rice and Tomatoes

Chinese Pork Puffs and Quick Stir-Fried Rice

Chinese Pan-Roasted Pork with Stir-Fried Bok Choy and Noodles

Dijon Pork with Red Pepper and Tomato Penne

Five-Spice Pork and Rice Stir-Fry

Ham and Lentil Soup with Country Garlic Toast

Herbed Grilled Pork with Tomato-Basil Pasta

Pan-Fried Pork with Garlic Greens with Spicy Roast Potatoes

Pork Chops with Apple Relish and Sweet Potatoes

Pork in Port Wine with Barley and Broccoli Rabe

Pork Medallions with Red Berry Sauce and Mixed-Herb Angel Hair Pasta

Pork Pita Pocket with Greek Salad

Roast Pork with Chunky Strawberry Salsa and Linguine with Summer Squash

Salsa Pork with Fresh Linguine

Sara Moulton's Pork Scaloppini with Broccoli and Sweet Potatoes

Southwestern Honey-Glazed Pork with Salsa Potato Salad

Whiskey Pork with Rosemary Lentils

BEEF   199

Beef in Oyster Sauce with Chinese Noodles

Buffalo Cheeseburgers with Mixed Salad

Filet Marchand de Vin (Steak in Red Wine Sauce) with Sautéed Garlic Potatoes

Garlic Steak with Chili Pepper Potatoes

Honey-Mustard Crusted Steak with Garlic Rosemary Beans

Meatball, Beer, and Potato Stew

Mediterranean Steak with Minted Couscous

Mock Hungarian Goulash with Caraway Noodles

Pan-Fried Ropa Vieja (Flank Steak in Tomato Sauce) and Brown Rice

Pistachio-Crusted Beef and Vegetable Kabobs

Roast Beef Chopped Salad

Roast Beef Hash with Mixed Green Salad

Roast Beef Pita Pocket with Tomato and Onion Relish and Greek Summer Salad

Spaghetti Bolognese (Spaghetti and Meat Sauce) with Herbed Zucchini

Steak and Portobello Sandwich with Tapenade-Topped Tomatoes

Walnut-Crusted Buffalo Steak with Tomato and Bean Salad

Vietnamese Hot and Spicy Stir-Fry Beef and Chinese Noodles with Snow Peas

VEAL & LAMB   235

Veal and Olive Stew with Quick Barley

Quick-Fried Diced Veal with Simple Fried Rice

Scaloppini al Marsala (Veal Marsala) with Penne ala Siciliana (Sicilian Penne Pasta)

Veal Milanese with Spaghettini Pomodoro

Veau aux Oranges (Veal in Orange Sauce) and Broccoli Rice Pilaf

Lamb and Lentil Tagine

Middle-Eastern Lamb with Spinach Brown Rice

VEGETARIAN   251

Frittata Primavera with Gratinéed Fennel

Greek-Style Casserole Soup

Indian-Spiced Spinach with Lentils and Rice

Mulligatawny Soup

Ricotta Soufflé with Tomato Bruschetta

Southwestern Three-Bean Soup

Tabbouleh with Toasted Walnut Couscous

Mushroom Pesto Pasta with Pimento Salad

INDEX   268

ACKNOWLEDGMENTS

One of the best parts of writing a book is working with so many talented and friendly people. I'd like to thank them all for their enthusiastic support.

My biggest thank you goes to my husband, Harold, who encouraged me, helped me test every recipe, and spent hours helping me edit every word. His constant encouragement for all of my work has made this book a partnership.

Thank you to Abe Ogden, Director of Book Publishing, and Greg Guthrie, Managing Editor, at the American Diabetes Association for their guidance and support. They worked closely with me to enable this book to come to life.

Thank you to my *Miami Herald* editor, Kathy Martin, for her constant support of my "Dinner in Minutes" column.

Thank you to Joseph Cooper, host of "Topical Currents," and to the staff at WLRN National Public Radio for their help and enthusiasm for my weekly "Food News and Views" segment.

I'd also like to thank my family, who have always supported my projects and encouraged me every step of the way: my son, James; his wife, Patty; and their children, Zachary, Jacob, and Haley; my son, John; his wife, Jill; and their children, Jeffrey and Joanna; and my son, Charles; his wife, Lori; and their sons, Daniel and Matthew; and my sister, Roberta, and brother-in-law Robert.

And finally, thank you to all of my readers and listeners who have written and called over the years. You have helped shape my ides and made the solitary task of writing a two-way street.

INTRODUCTION

Eating diabetes-friendly meals doesn't have to mean a lifestyle of steamed vegetables and broiled fish. Join me here for meals packed with flavor that can be made in minutes. Here's my secret. I let the supermarket do most of my preparation.

As a food writer, I find I am in the supermarket almost every day buying ingredients to test recipes. And now, what a pleasure—there are many advances that can help you in the kitchen without resorting to highly processed foods that are full of calories, fat, and salt.

My second secret is simple recipes packed with flavors. In this book, you will find a wide variety of ethnic dishes and some of your favorite comfort foods. Can I tempt you with **Braised Chinese Shrimp** (p. 54), **Indian-Spiced Chicken** (p. 126), **Southwestern Honey-Glazed Pork** (p. 194), and a comforting **Spaghetti Bolognese** (p. 226)?

Here's how this book will help you start on the quick, flavorful road to success.

SHOPPING

Less time spent in the supermarket is as important as cutting your kitchen time. To help speed you through the market, I've provided a shopping list with every dinner. I list the ingredients by departments—meat, grocery, produce, and dairy. Supermarkets are so large that forgetting something in the produce department when you're at the meat department can add time and frustration. All of the ingredients used in the recipes come from a local supermarket for one-stop shopping.

SHOP SMART!

Label reading takes time, and it's confusing to know what to look for. No more! Each meal in this book solves this problem. I give you the key nutritional information you need to look for on the prepared ingredients used in these recipes.

⚠ **SHOP SMART!** : use these as a guideline to find your favorite products. Stock them on your staples shelf for quick meals. Do you have to find the exact numbers? The answer here is no. Look for the products with the closest analysis.

STAPLES

In addition, I've included a list of the staples I call for in the recipes on page 5. Keeping staples on hand means that you only have to make a quick trip to the market for fresh ingredients.

HELPFUL HINTS AND COUNTDOWNS

Each dinner contains tips on shopping and cooking and a game plan, so you can get the whole meal on the table at the same time.

COOKING METHODS

Stir-Frying Make sure your wok is very hot. The oil should be smoking.

The secret to crisp, not steamed, stir-frying is to add the ingredients and let them sit for a minute before you toss them. The wok needs to regain its heat after the cold ingredients have been added.

For easy stir-frying, place the prepared ingredients on a cutting board or plate in the order you plan on using them. You won't have to look at the recipe once you start cooking.

Cooking Fish The general rule is to count 10 minutes for each inch of thickness. Fish continues to cook after it has been removed from the heat. I cook fish for 8 minutes per inch of thickness, remove it from the heat, and let it finish on its own.

To check for doneness, stick the point of a knife into the flesh. It should be opaque, not translucent.

Cooking Pasta Pasta should roll freely in plenty of boiling water. Use a very large pot and make sure the water is boiling. Add all of the pasta at one time and stir once.

SHOP SMART!

To help you get your dinner on the table in minutes, I have designed these recipes using many prepared ingredients that you can grab at your local grocery store. This guide isn't a specific recommendation for these products; you can choose from the many options available. The key is to ! SHOP SMART! by looking at the nutritional information I've highlighted for each item. Use these as a guideline for what you choose.

Many of these items can be added to your staples list, so you have them on hand for quick dinners.

DAIRY
Reduced-fat Mexican-style cheese, containing per ounce (1/4 cup): 80 calories, 5.5 g fat, 3.3 g saturated fat, 220 mg sodium

Low-fat cheddar cheese, containing per ounce: 49 calories, 2.0 g fat, 1.2 g saturated fat, 174 mg sodium

DELI
Low-fat ham, containing per ounce: 30 calories, 0.7 g fat, 0.2 g saturated fat, 301 mg sodium

Oven-roasted choice roast beef, no-salt-added, containing per ounce: 45 calories, 1.7 g fat, 0.8 g saturated fat, 20 mg sodium
Example: Boars Head brand

GROCERY
Reduced-fat pesto sauce, containing per tablespoon: 80 calories, 4.8 g total fat, 1 g saturated fat, 135 mg sodium
Example: Buitoni Reduced-fat Pesto with Basil

Low-sodium tomato juice, containing per cup (8 ounces): 41 calories, 10.3 g carbohydrate, 24 mg sodium

Low-sodium V8 juice, containing per cup (8 ounces): 51 calories, 10.0 g carbohydrate, 141 mg sodium

Sweet pickle relish, containing per tablespoon: 20 calories, 5.3 grams carbohydrate, 122 mg sodium

Chimichurri sauce, containing per tablespoon, 90 calories, 9.5 g fat, 33 mg sodium
Example: Badia Chimichurri Steak Sauce

Honey mustard, containing per tablespoon: 30 calories, 0 g fat, 15 mg sodium
Example: Grey Poupon

Fat-free refried beans, containing per 1/2 cup: 100 calories, 0 g fat, 580 mg sodium
Example: El Paso Fat-Free Refried Beans

Low-sodium teriyaki sauce, containing per tablespoon: 8 calories, 1.5 g carbohydrate, 168 mg sodium

Sweet and sour sauce, containing per tablespoon: 35 calories, 190 mg sodium
Example: Kikkoman brand

Thai peanut sauce, containing per tablespoon: 30 calories, 1.3 g fat, 3.2 g carbohydrate, 311 mg sodium
Example: Sanjay

Oyster sauce, containing per tablespoon: 9 calories, 492 mg sodium.

Organic vegetable broth, containing per cup: 12 calories, 3.0 g carbohydrate, 550 mg sodium

Reduced-fat vinaigrette or oil and vinegar dressing, containing per tablespoon: 11 calories, 1.0 g fat, 4 mg sodium

Low-sugar, low-sodium barbecue sauce, containing per tablespoon: 26 calories, 6.3 g carbohydrate, 23 mg sodium

Blue cheese creamy yogurt dressing, containing per 2 tablespoons: 50 calories, 4.5 g fat, 1.5 g saturated fat, 140 mg sodium
Example: Bold House Farms

Low-calorie Caesar salad dressing, containing per tablespoon: 16 calories, 0.7 g fat, 172 mg sodium

Canned sweet potatoes, containing per cup: 212 calories, 1.0 g fat, 50 g carbohydrate, 76 mg sodium

Canned potatoes, containing per cup: 112 calories, 0.36 g fat, 24.5 g carbohydrate, 9 mg sodium

Low-sodium canned whole tomatoes, containing per cup: 41 calories, 0.3 g fat, 9.6 g carbohydrate, 24 mg sodium

Canned low-sodium diced tomatoes, containing per cup: 41 calories, 9.6 g carbohydrate, 24 mg sodium

Canned crushed tomatoes, containing per cup: 41 calories, 0.3 g fat, 9.6 g carbohydrate, 24 mg sodium

Low-sodium tomato sauce, containing per cup (8 ounces): 103 calories, 0.5 g fat, 21.3 g carbohydrate, 21 mg sodium

Low-sodium pasta sauce, containing per 1/2 cup: 112 calories, 3.5 g fat, 17.7 g carbohydrate, 39 mg sodium

Canned lentils, containing per 1 cup: 240 calories, 680 mg sodium

Lite coconut milk, containing per 1/4 cup: 34 calories, 3.3 g fat, 1.9 g saturated fat, 2.3 g carbohydrate, 15 mg sodium

Salsa, containing per 2 tablespoons: 10 calories, 2 g carbohydrate, 65 mg sodium
Example: Newman's Own All-Natural Bandito Salsa

Black bean dip, containing per tablespoon: 15 calories, 0 fat, 2.5 g carbohydrate, 55 mg sodium

Sun-dried tomatoes in olive oil, containing per 2 teaspoons: 21 calories, 1.4 g fat, 2.3 g carbohydrate, 27 mg sodium

MEAT

Turkey sausage, containing per ounce: 44 calories, 2.2 g fat, 0.6 g saturated fat, 168 mg sodium

COOKING STAPLES

Keep these ingredients in your pantry or fridge and you will only have to pick up a few ingredients at the supermarket.

DAIRY
Eggs
Parmesan cheese

GROCERY
10-minute brown rice
Microwaveable brown rice
Long-grain white rice

SPICES
Salt
Black peppercorns
Dried oregano
Ground cumin
Ground ginger
Cayenne pepper
Dried thyme

BREADS
Whole-grain bread
Whole-wheat bread

CONDIMENTS
Reduced-fat mayonnaise
Hot pepper sauce
Lite soy sauce
Ketchup

OILS, VINEGARS, AND DRESSINGS
Olive oil
Canola oil
Balsamic vinegar
Distilled white vinegar
Olive oil spray
Reduced-fat vinaigrette dressing
Reduced-fat oil and vinegar dressing

MISCELLANEOUS
Sugar
Flour
Cornstarch
Bottled lemon juice
Frozen diced onion (or chopped)
Frozen diced green bell pepper (or chopped)
Frozen corn kernels
Canned potatoes
Fat-free, low-sodium chicken broth
Plain bread crumbs

PRODUCE
Minced garlic

SEAFOOD

Balsamic Grilled Tuna and Arugula Pasta 8

Texas Tuna Burger and Jalapeño Coleslaw 10

Hot Glazed Tuna Steak with Pecan Spinach Salad 12

Salmon, Quinoa, and Corn Salad 14

Chilled Cucumber and Salmon Soup 16

Poached Salmon with Chive Sauce and Vegetable Fettuccini 18

Salmon Gazpacho 20

Whiskey-Soused Salmon with Broccoli and Potatoes 22

Honey-Soy Glazed Salmon with Asparagus Rice 24

Almond-Crusted Trout with Penne and Sugar Snap Peas 26

Cumin-Crusted Snapper with Arroz con Jitomate (Rice with Tomato) 28

Sicilian Swordfish with Broccoli Linguine 30

Parmesan Sole with Dilled Potatoes 32

Fish in a Pouch with Garlic Couscous 34

Ginger-Teriyaki Steamed Fish and Chinese Noodles 36

Cajun-Bronzed Mahi-Mahi with Rice and Spinach Pilaf 38

Halibut in Cider with Saffron Rice 40

Five-Spice Fillet with Chinese Noodles and Sprouts 42

Southwestern Fish Fillet with Chipotle Corn and Zucchini 44

Pecan-Crusted Tilapia with Hot Pepper Succotash 46

Fish Chowder with Green Salad 48

Mexican Orange Fillet with Fried Corn and Green Pepper 50

Sautéed Fish with Pineapple Salsa and Poblano Rice 52

Braised Chinese Shrimp 54

Sweet and Sour Shrimp with Brown Rice 56

Spaghetti del Pescatore (Fisherman's Spaghetti) with Celery and Fennel Salad 58

Lemon-Pepper Shrimp and Couscous on a Bed of Spinach 60

Shrimp and Poblano Pepper Tacos with Pinto Bean Salad 62

Black Bean Soup with Shrimp 64

Shrimp Mushroom Quesadillas and Black Bean and Tomato Salad 66

Jerk Shrimp with Rice and Peas 68

Spicy Shrimp and Peach Salad with Lentils Vinaigrette 70

Hot Pepper Shrimp with Pimento Endive Salad 72

Shrimp Caesar Salad 74

Pan-Seared Scallops and Vegetable Medley Rice 76

Curry-Kissed Scallops with Carrots and Rice 78

Pesto Scallops with Fresh Fettuccini 80

Crab Scampi and Spaghetti 82

Spaghetti with Clams and Herb Sauce and Italian Salad 84

BALSAMIC GRILLED TUNA AND ARUGULA PASTA

Tuna steaks are a treat on the grill. The flavor varies with the different species of tuna. Yellowfin tuna, also known as ahi, is delicately flavored and works well for this recipe. I use a stove-top grill to make this dinner quickly.

Arugula is mostly used in cold salads. Anna, my Italian friend, likes to serve her arugula cooked, using it as the base for a pasta dish.

Balsamic Grilled Tuna

1/4 cup olive oil

2 tablespoons balsamic vinegar

1 teaspoon minced garlic

2 6-ounce tuna steaks, 3/4-inch thick (or one large steak)

COUNTDOWN

- ■ Marinate tuna.
- ■ Place water for pasta on stove to boil.
- ■ Prepare other ingredients.
- ■ Grill tuna.
- ■ Make pasta dish.

1. Mix the olive oil, balsamic vinegar, and garlic together in a plastic self-sealing bag or bowl.

2. Rinse the tuna, and add to the marinade. Let marinate 15 minutes, turning once during that time.

3. Drain tuna from marinade (only 2 tablespoons will be absorbed by the fish), and place on hot grill for 1 minute. Lift and make a quarter turn, leaving the tuna on the same side. This will help prevent the fish from sticking and make a cross-hatch pattern on the steak. Grill for 1 more minute, then turn over and leave 1 minute, lift and make a quarter turn and leave 1 minute for rare tuna. Grill 2 minutes longer for more well-done tuna. Remove from grill and serve.

Preparation time: 20 minutes ● Servings: 2

Calories 224 ● Calories from Fat 51 ● Total Fat 5.7 g ● Saturated Fat 1.0 g ● Monounsaturated Fat 3.2 g ● Cholesterol 78 mg ● Sodium 61 mg ● Carbohydrate 0.5 g ● Dietary Fiber 0 g ● Sugars 0.4 g ● Protein 39.8 ●

Exchanges: 5 lean meat

Arugula Pasta

1/4 pound fettuccini
1 1/2 tablespoons olive oil
6 cups washed ready-to-eat arugula
2 teaspoons minced garlic
2 tablespoons grated Parmesan cheese

1. Bring a large saucepan of water to a boil over high heat, and add fettucini. Cook 9 minutes if dried, or 2 minutes if fresh.
2. Heat olive oil in a skillet over medium-high heat, and add the arugula and garlic. Toss 1 minute. Add the drained pasta to the skillet, and toss all of the ingredients together.
3. Sprinkle Parmesan cheese on top. Remove from skillet and serve.

Preparation time: 10 minutes ● Servings: 2

Calories 346 ● Calories from Fat 116 ● Total Fat 12.9 g ● Saturated Fat 2.5 g ● Monounsaturated Fat 7.9 g ● Cholesterol 4 mg ● Sodium 96 mg ● Carbohydrate 46.9 g ● Dietary Fiber 2.9 g ● Sugars 2.9 g ● Protein 11.3 g

Exchanges: 3 starch, 1 vegetable, 2 fat

HELPFUL HINTS:

■ Marinate the tuna in a plastic self-sealing bag for easy clean up.
■ Any type of pasta can be used. Follow the cooking instructions on the package.

SHOPPING LIST

Seafood
2 6-ounce tuna steaks, 3/4-inch thick (or one large steak)

Dairy
1 small piece Parmesan cheese

Grocery
1/4 pound fettuccini

Produce
1 bag washed ready-to-eat arugula

Staples
Olive oil
Balsamic vinegar
Minced garlic

TEXAS TUNA BURGER AND JALAPEÑO COLESLAW

Fresh tuna seasoned with sweet pickle relish and scallions creates a tasty burger. Texans use peppers to add flavor to many of their dishes without adding too much heat. I have used hot pepper sauce in the burgers and jalapeño pepper in the coleslaw. Serve the coleslaw on the side or spoon some on top of the tuna burger.

Texas Tuna Burgers

2 whole-wheat hamburger rolls (2 ounces each)
2 scallions, thinly sliced
3/4 pound fresh tuna
1/4 cup sweet pickle relish **!**

Several drops hot pepper sauce
Salt
1 egg white
Olive oil spray

COUNTDOWN

■ Make coleslaw.
■ Toast hamburger rolls.
■ Prepare and cook tuna burgers.

1. Split hamburger rolls in half, and toast in toaster oven or under broiler until golden. Set aside.

2. Remove the stem end of the scallions, and break into three pieces. Chop in the food processor.

3. Add the tuna, pickle relish, hot pepper sauce, and salt to taste.

4. Remove from processor, and mix in egg white. Form into two burgers.

5. Heat a medium nonstick skillet over medium heat, and coat with with olive oil spray.

6. Add tuna burgers, and sauté 5 minutes; turn and sauté 3 more minutes. Serve on rolls.

Preparation time: 10 minutes ● Servings: 2

Calories 419 ● Calories from Fat 66 ● Total Fat 7.3 g ● Saturated Fat 1.3 g ● Monounsaturated Fat 3.0 g ● Cholesterol 78 mg ● Sodium 615 mg ● Carbohydrate 41.9 g ● Dietary Fiber 5.3 g ● Sugars 14.2 g ● Protein 47.0 g

Exchanges: 2 starch, 1/2 carbohydrate, 5 lean meat

Jalapeño Coleslaw

2 tablespoons reduced-fat mayonnaise
2 tablespoons distilled white vinegar
1 teaspoon sugar
2 medium jalapeño peppers, seeded and chopped (2 tablespoons)
Salt and freshly ground black pepper
1/2 cup fresh diced red onion
2 cups washed ready-to-eat, sliced cabbage

1. Mix mayonnaise, vinegar, sugar, and jalapeño pepper together in a medium bowl. Add salt and pepper to taste.
2. Add onion and cabbage. Toss well, making sure all of the cabbage is coated with the sauce. Set aside while tuna burgers cook.

Preparation time: 5 minutes ● Servings: 2

Calories 121 ● Calories from Fat 51 ● Total Fat 5.6 g ● Saturated Fat 0.9 g ● Monounsaturated Fat 1.3 g ● Cholesterol 5 mg ● Sodium 117 mg ● Carbohydrate 16.5 g ● Dietary Fiber 5.0 g ● Sugars 6.7 g ● Protein 2.7 g

Exchanges: 1 carbohydrate, 1 fat

HELPFUL HINTS:

■ Any type of fresh tuna can be used.

■ Diced fresh onions can be found in the produce section of the supermarket.

■ Seed jalapeño pepper and chop in a food processor. Remove and set aside.

■ Use the same food processor bowl, without washing it, to chop the scallions and then the tuna.

SHOPPING LIST

Seafood
3/4 pound fresh tuna

Grocery
1 package whole-wheat hamburger rolls
1 jar sweet pickle relish ⚠
1 bottle hot pepper sauce
1 bottle reduced-fat mayonnaise
1 bottle distilled white vinegar

Produce
1 bunch scallions
2 medium jalapeño peppers
1 container fresh diced red onion
1 bag washed ready-to-eat, sliced cabbage

Staples
Olive oil spray
Sugar
Egg
Salt
Black peppercorns

⚠ SHOP SMART!

Sweet pickle relish (per tablespoon): 20 calories, 5.3 grams carbohydrate, 122 mg sodium

HOT GLAZED TUNA STEAK WITH PECAN SPINACH SALAD

Fresh tuna steaks get a pleasing jolt from horseradish in this dish. It's slathered in a sweet and hot sauce that takes just minutes to make. Meaty and delicious, tuna steaks can dry out easily and need to be carefully cooked. It's best to undercook a little. The tuna will continue to cook after being removed from the stove.

Finish this quick meal with a salad of washed ready-to-eat spinach topped with grated carrots and pecans.

Hot Glazed Tuna Steak

2 1/2 tablespoons orange marmalade
1/2 tablespoon Dijon mustard
Several drops hot pepper sauce

1 teaspoon olive oil
3/4 pound fresh tuna steak
Salt and freshly ground black pepper

COUNTDOWN

◼ Make salad.
◼ Make tuna.

1. Mix together marmalade and mustard. Add a few drops hot pepper sauce. Set aside. Heat oil in a medium nonstick skillet over medium-high heat.

2. Sear tuna for 2 minutes. Turn and sprinkle salt and pepper on the cooked side. Sear second side 2 minutes for a 1/2-inch-thick tuna steak. For a 1-inch tuna steak, lower heat and cook 2 more minutes.

3. Transfer to individual dinner plates. Add marmalade mixture to skillet, and sauté 30 seconds or until marmalade melts, scraping up any brown bits in the pan.

4. Spoon sauce over tuna. Serve.

Preparation time: 10 minutes ● Servings: 2

Calories 276 ● Calories from Fat 36 ● Total Fat 4.0 g ● Saturated Fat 0.7 g ● Monounsaturated Fat 2.0 g ● Cholesterol 78 mg ● Sodium 114 mg ● Carbohydrate 17.7 g ● Dietary Fiber 0.1 g ● Sugars 0 g ● Protein 40.1 g

Exchanges: 1 carbohydrate, 5 lean meat

Pecan Spinach Salad

5 cups washed ready-to-eat baby spinach (about 5 ounces)
2 cups shredded carrots (about 3 ounces)
1/2 cup broken unsalted pecans (1 3/4 ounces)
2 tablespoons reduced-fat vinaigrette dressing ⚠
Salt and freshly ground black pepper

1. Place spinach on individual dinner plates.
2. Spoon carrots and pecans onto spinach. Add dressing, and toss well.
3. Season with salt and pepper to taste. Serve.

Preparation time: 5 minutes ● Servings: 2

Calories 245 ● Calories from Fat 175 ● Total Fat 19.4 g ● Saturated Fat 1.7 g ● Monounsaturated Fat 10.5 g ● Cholesterol 1 mg ● Sodium 140 mg ● Carbohydrate 17.4 g ● Dietary Fiber 7.2 g ● Sugars 7.2 g ● Protein 5.5 g

Exchanges: 1/2 carbohydrate, 2 vegetable, 3 1/2 fat

HELPFUL HINTS:

■ Shredded carrots, sometimes called matchstick carrots, are available in the produce section of the market.

■ If baby spinach is not available, use regular spinach and tear into bite-size pieces.

SHOPPING LIST

Seafood
3/4 pound fresh tuna steak

Grocery
1 jar orange marmalade
1 jar Dijon mustard
1 small bottle hot pepper sauce
1 small package unsalted broken pecans

Produce
1 bag washed ready-to-eat baby spinach
1 bag shredded carrots

Staples
Olive oil
Reduced-fat vinaigrette dressing ⚠
Salt
Black peppercorns

⚠ **SHOP SMART!**

Reduced-fat vinaigrette or oil and vinegar dressing (per tablespoon): 11 calories, 1.0 g fat, 4 mg sodium

SALMON, QUINOA, AND CORN SALAD

Salmon, quinoa, and corn are typical Chilean ingredients. Here they are combined to make a quick salad supper.

Quinoa is an ancient grain that is indigenous to the Andes Mountains in South America. It's considered a superfood because it contains more protein than any other grain and is a good source of fiber. It can be cooked like rice.

Using frozen corn, frozen lima beans, and diced tomatoes from the produce section of the market helps make this dinner a breeze.

Salmon, Quinoa, and Corn Salad

2 cups water
1/2 cup frozen corn kernels
1/2 cup quinoa, rinsed in cold water
1/4 cup frozen lima beans
1 cup fresh diced tomato
1 teaspoon ground cumin

2 tablespoons reduced-fat vinaigrette dressing ⚡
Salt and freshly ground black pepper
Olive oil spray
3/4 pound wild-caught salmon fillet
1 cup washed ready-to-eat spinach
2 tablespoons chopped cilantro (optional)

COUNTDOWN

■ Prepare the ingredients.
■ Start the quinoa cooking.
■ While the quinoa cooks, sauté the salmon.

1. Place water, corn, quinoa, and lima beans in a saucepan and bring to a boil. Cook, uncovered, 10 minutes or until quinoa soaks up the liquid and becomes soft.

2. Remove from the heat, add the tomato, and sprinkle cumin on top. Add the vinaigrette and salt and pepper to taste. Toss well and set aside.

3. While quinoa cooks, heat a small nonstick skillet over medium-high heat. Spray with olive oil spray, and add the salmon. Sauté 4 minutes; turn and sauté 4 minutes. Add salt and pepper to taste.

4. To serve, arrange spinach leaves on two dinner plates. Divide the salmon in half, and place on the plates over the spinach. Sprinkle chopped cilantro (optional) over salmon. Serve with quinoa and corn salad.

Preparation time: 15 minutes ● Servings: 2

Calories 510 ● Calories from Fat 140 ● Total Fat 15.5 g ● Saturated Fat 2.3 g ● Monounsaturated Fat 5.4 g ● Cholesterol 97 mg ● Sodium 139 mg ● Carbohydrate 46.9 g ● Dietary Fiber 6.5 g ● Sugars 5.4 g ● Protein 48.6 g

Exchanges: 3 starch, 5 lean meat, 1 fat

HELPFUL HINTS:

- Quinoa can be found in the grain section of most supermarkets.
- Diced fresh tomatoes can be found in the produce section of the supermarket.
- The salmon can be served at room temperature or warm over the salad.
- A quick way to chop cilantro is to snip the leaves with scissors.

SHOPPING LIST

Seafood
3/4 pound wild-caught salmon fillet

Grocery
1 package quinoa
1 jar ground cumin
1 package frozen lima beans
1 package frozen corn kernels

Produce
1 container fresh diced tomato
1 package washed ready-to-eat
   spinach
1 small bunch cilantro (*optional*)

Staples
Olive oil spray
Reduced-fat vinaigrette *!*
Salt
Black peppercorns

! SHOP SMART!

Reduced-fat vinaigrette or oil and vinegar dressing (per tablespoon): 11 calories, 1.0 g fat, 4 mg sodium

CHILLED CUCUMBER AND SALMON SOUP

This frothy soup made with cucumbers, onion, dill, and sautéed fresh salmon makes a soothing summer supper. The contrast between the textures and tastes brings out the full flavor of the salmon.

Chilled Cucumber and Salmon Soup

2 teaspoons olive oil
3/4 pound wild-caught salmon fillet
3 cups fresh diced cucumber, divided
1 cup frozen diced onion
1/2 cup clam juice
1 cup water
1 cup nonfat plain yogurt

2 teaspoons dried dill
Salt and freshly ground black pepper

Garnish
2 scallions, sliced
2 slices whole-grain bread

COUNTDOWN

■ Prepare
   ingredients.
■ Cook salmon.
■ Complete soup.

1. Heat olive oil in a medium saucepan over medium-high heat. Add salmon and sauté 3 minutes; turn and sauté 3 minutes for a 3/4-inch piece or until salmon is cooked through. If the salmon is thicker, cook another 1 minute per side.

2. Transfer to two large soup bowls. Cut into 2-inch slices. Set aside.

3. Set aside 2 tablespoons diced cucumber; add remainder to the saucepan, along with the onion, clam juice, and water. Bring to a simmer, cover with a lid, and cook until cucumbers are soft, about 5 minutes.

4. Place in a blender or food processor, and add the yogurt and dill. Blend until smooth. Add salt and pepper to taste.

5. To serve, pour soup over the salmon slices in the two soup bowls. Sprinkle reserved cucumber and scallions on top. Serve with bread.

Preparation time: 15 minutes ● Servings: 2

Calories 484 ● Calories from Fat 142 ● Total Fat 15.8 g ● Saturated Fat 2.6 g ● Monounsaturated Fat 6.6 g ● Cholesterol 99 mg ● Sodium 588 mg ● Carbohydrate 35.4 g ● Dietary Fiber 4.9 g ● Sugars 7.9 g ● Protein 51.4 g

Exchanges: 1 starch, 1/2 fat-free milk, 2 vegetable, 5 lean meat, 1 1/2 fat

HELPFUL HINTS:

■ Salmon fillets or steak can be used.

■ Fresh diced cucumber is available in the produce section of the supermarket. If unavailable, use fresh cucumber.

■ Fresh dill can be used instead of dried.

POACHED SALMON WITH CHIVE SAUCE AND VEGETABLE FETTUCCINI

A light chive sauce tops gently poached salmon fillets in this quick dinner. Fresh fettucini with carrots and broccoli complete this simple, elegant meal.

Shredded carrots can be found in the produce section of the supermarket, along with broccoli florets. This means there's no slicing and chopping for the Vegetable Fettuccini side dish.

Poached Salmon with Chive Sauce

3/4 pound wild-caught salmon fillet, skin removed
2 teaspoons olive oil
1/2 tablespoon bottled lemon juice

3 tablespoons snipped fresh chives or
   1 tablespoon freeze-dried chives
Salt and freshly ground black pepper

COUNTDOWN

■ Place water for pasta on to boil.
■ Make salmon.
■ While salmon poaches, make pasta.

1. Bring a medium saucepan full of water to a boil over high heat.
2. Lower the heat to medium-low, and add the salmon fillet. The salmon should be completely covered by the water, and the water should be at a gentle simmer. Simmer the salmon for 3 minutes. Remove from the heat, and let the salmon rest in the liquid for 3 minutes for a 1-inch-thick piece of salmon.
3. Mix the olive oil, lemon juice, and chives together.
4. Remove the salmon from the poaching liquid. Sprinkle with salt and pepper to taste. Spoon the sauce over the salmon. Serve.

Preparation time: 10 minutes ● Servings: 2

Calories 288 ● Calories from Fat 126 ● Total Fat 14.0 g ● Saturated Fat 2.2 g ● Monounsaturated Fat 6.3 g ● Cholesterol 96 mg ● Sodium 96 mg ● Carbohydrate 2.6 g ● Dietary Fiber 0.2 g ● Sugars 0.2 g ● Protein 38.6 g

Exchanges: 5 lean meat, 1 1/2 fat

Vegetable Fettuccini

1/4 pound fresh whole-wheat fettuccini
2 cups shredded carrots
1 cup broccoli florets
1 tablespoon olive oil
Salt and freshly ground black pepper

1. Bring a large saucepan with 3–4 quarts of water to a boil over high heat.
2. Add the fettuccini, carrots, and broccoli florets. Bring back to a boil, and cook 4–5 minutes.
3. Remove about 2 tablespoons of the cooking water and set aside. Drain the pasta. Add the reserved water, olive oil, salt and pepper to taste. Toss well. Serve.

Preparation time: 10 minutes ● Servings: 2

Calories 313 ● Calories from Fat 71 ● Total Fat 7.9 g ● Saturated Fat 1.1 g ● Monounsaturated Fat 5.1 g ● Cholesterol 0 mg ● Sodium 91mg ● Carbohydrate 55.2 g ● Dietary Fiber 7.8 g ● Sugars 7.3 g ● Protein 10.4 g

Exchanges: 3 starch, 1 vegetable, 1 fat

HELPFUL HINTS:

■ Any type of vegetable can be used for the fettuccini. Try sliced daikon or white radish for a slight bite to the pasta.

■ Fresh lemon juice can be used instead of bottled.

■ Any type of whole-wheat pasta can be used. Follow package instructions for cooking and add the vegetables 3 minutes before pasta is ready for draining.

■ A quick way to slice chives is to snip them with scissors.

■ The cooking method is for a 1-inch salmon fillet. Reduce or add the resting time depending on the size of your fillet. Let the salmon rest for 2 minutes for a 1/2-inch thick salmon or for 4 minutes for a 1 1/2- to 2-inch thick fillet.

SHOPPING LIST

Seafood
3/4 pound wild-caught salmon fillet

Grocery
1/4 pound fresh whole-wheat fettuccini
1 bottle lemon juice

Produce
1 bag shredded carrots
1 small package broccoli florets
1 bunch fresh chives

Staples
Olive oil
Salt
Black peppercorns

SALMON GAZPACHO

Fresh salmon, cucumbers, and tomatoes make a tasty combination in this creamy soup supper. Gazpacho is a Spanish soup served at room temperature or chilled. Adding freshly cooked salmon creates a complete one-dish meal in which the soup ingredients flavor the salmon.

The secret to the rich flavor of this dinner is that the salmon is cooked for just a few minutes on its own and removed from the saucepan, so that it does not overcook. It's then added to the remaining ingredients in the gazpacho so the flavors can blend.

The salmon may be a little red in the center when it is removed from the skillet. It will continue to cook in its own heat once it is removed.

Salmon Gazpacho

3/4 pound wild-caught salmon fillet

1 cup low-sodium tomato juice ⚡

2 cups plus 2 tablespoons fresh diced tomatoes, divided

3/4 cup fresh diced onion

3/4 cup plus 2 tablespoons fresh diced cucumber, divided

2 teaspoons olive oil

2 teaspoons balsamic vinegar

1 cup nonfat plain yogurt

Salt and freshly ground black pepper

2 slices crusty whole-wheat bread

2 scallions, sliced

COUNTDOWN

■ Prepare ingredients.
■ Cook salmon.
■ Toast bread.
■ Complete soup.

1. Heat a nonstick skillet over medium-high heat. Add the salmon and sauté 3 minutes; turn and sauté 3 minutes for a 3/4-inch piece. If the salmon is thicker, cook another 2 minutes per side until salmon is cooked through.

2. While salmon cooks, pour tomato juice into a blender or food processor. Add 2 cups tomatoes, the onion, 3/4 cup diced cucumber, olive oil, balsamic vinegar, and yogurt.

3. Blend until smooth. Add salt and pepper to taste.

4. Divide between 2 large soup bowls.

5. Toast bread.

6. Cut cooked salmon into 1- to 2-inch pieces, and divide between the bowls.

7. Sprinkle remaining 2 tablespoons diced tomatoes and 2 tablespoons diced cucumber over soup, and sprinkle scallions on top. Serve with a slice of bread.

Preparation time: 15 minutes ● Servings: 2

Calories 518 ● Calories from Fat 142 ● Total Fat 15.8 g ● Saturated Fat 2.6 g ● Monounsaturated Fat 6.9 g ● Cholesterol 98.5 mg ● Sodium 351 mg ● Carbohydrate 44.6 g ● Dietary Fiber 6.5 g ● Sugars 15.4 g ● Protein 53.0 g

Exchanges: 1 starch, 1/2 fat-free milk, 3 vegetable, 6 lean meat, 1 fat

HELPFUL HINTS:

■ Salmon fillets or steak can be used.

■ Low-sodium V8 juice can be used instead of low-sodium tomato juice.

■ Fresh diced tomatoes, cucumber, and onion can be found in the produce section of the supermarket.

■ A quick way to slice scallions is to snip them with scissors.

WHISKEY-SOUSED SALMON WITH BROCCOLI AND POTATOES

A light whiskey-flavored mayonnaise sauce dresses the salmon steaks in this wonderful supper. Potatoes and broccoli, livened with chives, can be made in minutes in a microwave oven.

Salmon is sold in thick steaks with the bone in or in thin fillets. The steaks are a nice alternative to the fillets.

Whiskey-Soused Salmon

2 6-ounce wild-caught salmon steaks
Salt and freshly ground black pepper
Olive oil spray
2 tablespoons reduced-fat mayonnaise

1 tablespoon lemon juice
1 tablespoon whiskey
Several sprigs of watercress (*optional*)

COUNTDOWN

■ Preheat broiler
■ Start salmon.
■ Make salmon sauce.
■ Make potatoes.
■ Finish salmon.

1. Preheat broiler. Line a baking tray with foil, and add salmon steaks.
2. Sprinkle with salt and pepper to taste. Spray olive oil on top.
3. Broil 6 inches from heat for 5 minutes. Turn and broil 4 minutes more.
4. Meanwhile, mix mayonnaise, lemon juice, and whiskey together. Place salmon on dinner plates and spoon sauce on top.
5. Garnish with watercress (*optional*). Serve.

Preparation time: 10 minutes ● Servings: 2

Calories 330 ● Calories from Fat 143 ● Total Fat 15.9 g ● Saturated Fat 2.5 g ● Monounsaturated Fat 5.3 g ● Cholesterol 101 mg ● Sodium 199 mg ● Carbohydrate 4.4 g ● Dietary Fiber 0 g ● Sugars 0.8 g ● Protein 38.6 g

Exchanges: 5 lean meat, 2 fat

Broccoli and Potatoes

3/4 pound canned potatoes (about 2 cups), rinsed and drained
1/2 pound broccoli florets (about 3 cups)
1 tablespoon olive oil
1/2 tablespoon dried chives
Salt and freshly ground black pepper

1. Cut drained potatoes into 3/4- to 1-inch pieces.
2. Cut broccoli florets in half. Place in a microwave-safe bowl, and microwave on high 2 minutes.
3. Remove and add olive oil, chives, and salt and pepper to taste. Gently toss, being careful not to break up the potatoes. Serve.

Preparation time: 5 minutes ● Servings: 2

Calories 212 ● Calories from Fat 67 ● Total Fat 7.4 g ● Saturated Fat 1.0 g
● Monounsaturated Fat 5.0 g ● Cholesterol 0 mg ● Sodium 41 mg ●
Carbohydrate 33.1g ● Dietary Fiber 2.9 g ● Sugars 1.7 g ● Protein 6.6 g

Exchanges: 1 1/2 starch, 2 vegetable, 1 fat

HELPFUL HINTS:

■ If you prefer not to use whiskey in the sauce, 2 tablespoons of tomato paste can be used instead.

■ Salmon fillets can be used.

SHOPPING LIST

Seafood
2 6-ounce wild-caught salmon steaks

Grocery
2 14.5-ounce cans whole potatoes
1 bottle reduced-fat mayonnaise
1 bottle lemon juice
1 small bottle whiskey
1 bottle dried chives

Produce
1 bunch watercress (*optional*)
1/2 pound broccoli florets

Staples
Olive oil spray
Olive oil
Salt
Black peppercorns

HONEY-SOY GLAZED SALMON WITH ASPARAGUS RICE

Add a savory, sweet flavor to salmon with this honey-soy glaze. Roasting in the oven intensifies the flavor of the ingredients but takes much longer than sautéing. Pan-roasting is a great compromise. The salmon fillet is sautéed and then roasted in a covered skillet for 7–8 minutes for a 3/4-inch fillet.

Honey-Soy Glazed Salmon

3/4 pound wild-caught salmon fillet
Olive oil spray
Salt and freshly ground black pepper

1 tablespoon honey
1 tablespoon reduced-sodium soy sauce

COUNTDOWN

■ Place water for rice on to boil.
■ Prepare remaining ingredients.
■ Make rice.
■ While rice cooks, make salmon.

1. Rinse salmon and pat dry with a paper towel.
2. Heat a nonstick skillet over medium-high heat, and spray with olive oil spray.
3. Brown salmon 2 minutes; turn and brown 1 minute. Season the cooked sides with salt and pepper. Lower heat to low, cover, and let cook 7–8 minutes. Remove from heat.
4. Mix honey and soy sauce together. Pour over the salmon, cover, and let sit 1 minute. Serve.

Preparation time: 15 minutes ● Servings: 2

Calories 303 ● Calories from Fat 105 ● Total Fat 11.6 g ● Saturated Fat 1.9 g ● Monounsaturated Fat 4.6 g ● Cholesterol 96 mg ● Sodium 366 mg ● Carbohydrate 12 g ● Dietary Fiber 0.1 g ● Sugars 8.8 g ● Protein 38.9 g

Exchanges: 1 carbohydrate, 5 lean meat, 1/2 fat

Asparagus Rice

1/2 pound asparagus, cut into 1-inch pieces (about 2 cups)
2 cups water
1 cup 10-minute brown rice (to make 1 1/2 cups cooked rice)
1 tablespoon olive oil
Salt and freshly ground black pepper

1. Wash asparagus, and cut off hard ends and discard. Cut into 1-inch pieces.
2. Add water to a saucepan, and bring to a boil over high heat. Add rice and asparagus. Cover with a lid, and boil 5 minutes.
3. Remove from heat. Let sit 5 minutes.
4. Toss with olive oil and salt and pepper to taste. Serve.

Preparation time: 12 minutes ● Servings: 2

Calories 241 ● Calories from Fat 77 ● Total Fat 8.5 g ● Saturated Fat 1.3 g ● Monounsaturated Fat 5.4 g ● Cholesterol 0 mg ● Sodium 13 mg ● Carbohydrate 40.1g ● Dietary Fiber 4.8 g ● Sugars 0 g ● Protein 6.1 g

Exchanges: 2 starch, 1 vegetable, 1 1/2 fat

HELPFUL HINTS:

■ If salmon gives off oil when it is cooked, pour the oil off before adding the glaze.

SHOPPING LIST

Seafood
3/4 pound wild-caught salmon fillet

Grocery
1 small bottle reduced-sodium
   soy sauce
1 small jar honey
1 box 10-minute brown rice

Produce
1/2 pound asparagus

Staples
Olive oil spray
Olive oil
Salt
Black peppercorns

ALMOND-CRUSTED TROUT WITH PENNE AND SUGAR SNAP PEAS

Fresh trout topped with toasted almonds takes only minutes to make. Whole farm-raised trout is available in many markets. If you prefer, ask for the head and tail to be removed and for the fish to be filleted.

Toasting almonds intensifies their flavor. This can be done in a toaster oven or under a broiler.

Almond-Crusted Trout

1/4 cup sliced almonds (1 ounce)
2 whole trout, about 1/2 pound each, heads and tails removed, filleted

Salt and freshly ground black pepper
Olive oil spray
2 tablespoons chopped parsley (*optional*)

COUNTDOWN

- Place water for pasta on to boil.
- Prepare ingredients.
- Toast the almonds.
- Cook the pasta.
- While pasta cooks, sauté the trout.

1. Heat a nonstick skillet over medium-high heat. Add almonds and toast 1 minute or until golden. Transfer to a plate.
2. Open trout flat. Season with salt and pepper to taste.
3. Raise the heat to high, spray skillet with olive oil spray, and place trout skin side down in skillet. Sauté 4 minutes; turn and sauté 2 minutes.
4. Transfer to two dinner plates, and scatter almond crust over trout. Sprinkle parsley on top (if desired).

Preparation time: 10 minutes ● Servings: 2

Calories 352 ● Calories from Fat 188 ● Total Fat 20.9 g ● Saturated Fat 2.7 g ● Monounsaturated Fat 11.9 g ● Cholesterol 88 mg ● Sodium 92 mg ● Carbohydrate 4.2 g ● Dietary Fiber 2.0 g ● Sugars 0.9 g ● Protein 36.4 g

Exchanges: 5 lean meat, 2 1/2 fat

Penne and Sugar Snap Peas

1/4 pound whole-grain penne pasta
1/2 pound sugar snap peas, trimmed (about 3 3/4 cups)
2 teaspoons olive oil
2 tablespoons lemon juice
Salt and freshly ground black pepper

1. Bring a large saucepan with 3–4 quarts of water to a boil.

2. Add penne pasta, and boil 7 minutes.

3. Add the sugar snap peas. Continue to boil 2–3 minutes or until pasta is cooked al dente.

4. Drain, leaving about 1 tablespoon cooking water on the pasta. Toss with olive oil, lemon juice, and salt and pepper to taste. Serve on plates with trout.

Preparation time: 15 minutes ● Servings: 2

Calories 303 ● Calories from Fat 50 ● Total Fat 5.6 g ● Saturated Fat 0.8 g ● Monounsaturated Fat 3.4 g ● Cholesterol 0 mg ● Sodium 8 mg ● Carbohydrate 52.5 g ● Dietary Fiber 4.8 g ● Sugars 6.4 g ● Protein 10.7 g

Exchanges: 3 starch, 1 vegetable, 1 fat

HELPFUL HINTS:

■ If trout is not available, use any type of fish fillet (tilapia, grouper, mahi-mahi, flounder, or sole). Measure the fish at its thickest part and cook for 10 minutes per inch of thickness.

■ Green beans or snow peas can be used instead of sugar snap peas.

■ Any short cut pasta can be used.

SHOPPING LIST

Seafood
2 whole trout, about 1/2 pound each, heads and tails removed, filleted

Grocery
1 ounce sliced almonds
1 small package whole-grain penne pasta
1 bottle lemon juice

Produce
1 bunch parsley (*optional*)
1/2 pound trimmed sugar snap peas

Staples
Olive oil spray
Olive oil
Salt
Black peppercorns

CUMIN-CRUSTED SNAPPER WITH ARROZ CON JITOMATE (RICE WITH TOMATO)

A coating of cumin flavors the firm-textured, slightly sweet snapper in this simple Latin meal. I had some leftovers and found that the fish was delicious when served at room temperature the next day. If you have time, make extra for another quick meal or lunch.

Arroz con Jitomate (or rice with tomato) is a Mexican rice dish traditionally made with fresh, ripe tomatoes that have been peeled and mashed. Using organic, canned diced tomatoes gives a fresh flavor without the time-consuming work.

Cumin-Crusted Snapper

2 tablespoons flour
2 teaspoons ground cumin
Salt and freshly ground black pepper

3/4 pound snapper fillets, skin removed
1 egg white, lightly beaten
1 tablespoon canola oil

COUNTDOWN

■ Start rice.
■ Prepare ingredients.
■ Make fish.
■ Finish rice.

1. Mix together flour, cumin, and salt and pepper to taste in a bowl. Set aside.

2. Dip snapper fillet in the egg white and then in the flour mixture. Coat both sides of the fillet and shake off extra flour.

3. Heat the oil in a nonstick skillet over medium-high heat. Sauté 3 minutes; turn and sauté 5 minutes. Test to see if the fish is ready. Spread the flesh aside with the tip of a knife. The flesh should be opaque and not translucent. Serve.

Preparation time: 10 minutes ● Servings: 2

Calories 272 ● Calories from Fat 86 ● Total Fat 9.6 g ● Saturated Fat 1.0 g ● Monounsaturated Fat 5.0 g ● Cholesterol 60 mg ● Sodium 140 mg ● Carbohydrate 7.0 g ● Dietary Fiber 0.4 g ● Sugars 0.1g ● Protein 37.8 g

Exchanges: 1/2 starch, 5 lean meat

Arroz con Jitomate (Rice with Tomato)

1 package microwaveable brown rice (to make 1 1/2 cups cooked rice)
1 cup sliced green bell pepper
1 cup drained, canned low-sodium diced tomatoes ❗
2 teaspoons canola oil
Salt and freshly ground black pepper
2 tablespoons chopped fresh cilantro (*optional*)

1. Cook brown rice according to package instructions in the microwave. Measure 1 1/2 cups cooked rice and reserve remaining rice for another meal.

2. Place green bell pepper slices in a bowl and microwave on high 1 minute. Remove the bowl from the microwave. Add the rice, tomatoes, oil, and salt and pepper to taste to the bowl. Toss well.

3. Sprinkle cilantro on top (if desired).

Preparation time: 5 minutes ● Servings: 2

Calories 251 ● Calories from Fat 66 ● Total Fat 7.4 g ● Saturated Fat 0.8 g ● Monounsaturated Fat 3.6 g ● Cholesterol 0 mg ● Sodium 18 mg ● Carbohydrate 36.3 g ● Dietary Fiber 3.9 g ● Sugars 4.2 g ● Protein 5.2 g

Exchanges: 2 starch, 1 vegetable, 1 1/2 fat

HELPFUL HINTS:

■ Any type of white-fleshed fish fillet, such as tilapia, grouper, or pompano, can be used.

■ If you want more kick to the rice, add several drops of hot pepper sauce to the diced tomatoes.

SHOPPING LIST

Seafood
3/4 pound snapper fillets, skin removed

Grocery
1 jar ground cumin
1 package microwaveable brown rice
1 14.5-ounce can low-sodium diced tomatoes ❗

Produce
1 medium green bell pepper
1 bunch cilantro (*optional*)

Staples
Flour
Egg
Canola oil
Salt
Black peppercorns

❗ SHOP SMART!

Canned low-sodium diced tomatoes (per cup): 41 calories, 9.6 g carbohydrate, 24 mg sodium

SICILIAN SWORDFISH WITH BROCCOLI LINGUINE

Tomatoes, olives, and garlic are staples in zesty Sicilian cooking. Raisins add sweetness, giving the sauce in this dish a tantalizing sweet and sour flavor. The sauce for the fish can be made in a microwave oven. This saves time and the need to clean another saucepan. There is also a stove-top method.

Sicilian Swordfish

1 cup canned, drained, low-sodium diced tomatoes ⚡
2 teaspoons minced garlic
5 pitted black olives
2 tablespoons raisins

1 teaspoon dried oregano
Salt and freshly ground black pepper
1 teaspoon olive oil
3/4 pound swordfish (about 3/4 inch thick)

For sauce:

Microwave method: Place tomatoes, garlic, olives, raisins, and oregano in a microwave-safe bowl. Cover with a paper towel, and microwave on high 2 minutes. Add salt and pepper to taste.

Stove method: Place tomatoes and garlic in a small saucepan, and simmer 2 minutes. Add olives, raisins, and oregano, and continue to cook 5 minutes. Add salt and pepper to taste.

COUNTDOWN

■ Place water for pasta on to boil.
■ Cook sauce and then fish.
■ Boil pasta

For fish:

1. Heat olive oil in a medium nonstick skillet over medium-high heat.
2. Add swordfish. Brown for 2 minutes; turn and brown for 2 minutes. Season cooked sides with salt and pepper.
3. Lower heat to medium, and continue to cook 1 minute for 3/4-inch-thick fish or 2 minutes for 1-inch-thick fish. It will look opaque inside, not translucent.
4. Remove from skillet. Divide into two equal portions. Serve over linguine. Spoon sauce over top.

Preparation time: 10 minutes ● Servings: 2

Calories 291 ● Calories from Fat 92 ● Total Fat 10.2 g ● Saturated Fat 2.5 g ● Monounsaturated Fat 4.9 g ● Cholesterol 66 mg ● Sodium 241 mg ● Carbohydrate 14.8 g ● Dietary Fiber 2.2 g ● Sugars 8.3 g ● Protein 35.4 g

Exchanges: 1 carbohydrate, 5 lean meat

Broccoli Linguine

1/4 pound fresh whole-wheat linguine
1/4 pound broccoli florets (about 1 1/2 cups)
2 teaspoons olive oil
Salt and freshly ground black pepper

1. Bring a large saucepan with 3 quarts of water to a boil over high heat. Add linguine and broccoli. Cook 3 minutes if using fresh pasta. If using dried linguine, boil 6 minutes.

2. Add broccoli, and boil 3 more minutes.

3. Transfer 2 tablespoons water from saucepan to a bowl. Mix olive oil into water in bowl.

4. Drain linguine and broccoli, and add to the bowl.

5. Add salt and pepper to taste. Place on individual plates. Serve fish and sauce over pasta.

Preparation time: 10 minutes ● Servings: 2

Calories 267 ● Calories from Fat 50 ● Total Fat 5.6 g ● Saturated Fat 0.8 g ● Monounsaturated Fat 3.4 g ● Cholesterol 0 mg ● Sodium 18 mg ● Carbohydrate 45.5 g ● Dietary Fiber 1.8 g ● Sugars 1.5 g ● Protein 9 g

Exchanges: 2 1/2 starch, 1 vegetable, 1 fat

SHOPPING LIST

Seafood
3/4 pound swordfish
  (about 3/4-inch thick)

Grocery
1 can low-sodium diced tomatoes ❗
1 can pitted black olives
1 small box raisins
1 bottle dried oregano
1 package fresh whole-wheat
  linguine

Produce
1/4 pound broccoli florets

Staples
Olive oil
Minced garlic
Salt
Black peppercorns

❗ SHOP SMART!

Canned low-sodium diced tomatoes (per cup): 41 calories, 9.6 g carbohydrate, 24 mg sodium

HELPFUL HINTS:

■ Any meaty type of fish, such as tuna, halibut, or grouper, can be used.

■ If using dried pasta instead of fresh, cook it for 9 minutes or according to package directions.

■ Minced garlic can be found in jars in the produce section of the supermarket.

PARMESAN SOLE WITH DILLED POTATOES

Using fresh fish and canned potatoes, this meal can be ready to eat in less than 15 minutes. For the best flavor, the fish should be very fresh. Buy whatever looks best that day. Also look for good-quality Parmigiano-Reggiano.

Parmesan Sole

Olive oil spray

3/4 pound sole fillets (or thin white fish fillet about 1/2-inch thick)

Salt and freshly ground black pepper

1 medium tomato, sliced (about 1 cup)

3 tablespoons grated Parmesan cheese

1 teaspoon dried oregano

COUNTDOWN

■ Start fish.
■ While fish cooks, microwave potatoes.

1. Heat a large nonstick skillet over medium-high heat, and spray with olive oil spray. Add fish fillets in one layer. Sprinkle with salt and pepper to taste.

2. Arrange tomato slices over fillets. Spread Parmesan cheese on top, and sprinkle with oregano. Cover with a lid, and sauté 5 minutes. Remove from skillet and serve.

Preparation time: 7 minutes ● Servings: 2

Calories 221 ● Calories from Fat 53 ● Total Fat 5.8 g ● Saturated Fat 2.2 g ● Monounsaturated Fat 2.1 g ● Cholesterol 90 mg ● Sodium 259 mg ● Carbohydrate 4.5 g ● Dietary Fiber 1.3 g ● Sugars 2.5 g ● Protein 35.8 g

Exchanges: 5 lean meat, 1 vegetable

Dilled Potatoes

1 pound canned potatoes, rinsed and drained (about 2 1/2 cups) ⚡
4 teaspoons olive oil
1/2 tablespoon dried dill
Salt and freshly ground black pepper

1. Cut drained potatoes into 3/4- to 1-inch pieces.

2. Place in a microwave-safe bowl, and microwave on high 2 minutes.

3. Remove. Add olive oil, dried dill, and salt and pepper to taste. Gently toss, being careful not to break up the potatoes. Serve.

Preparation time: 5 minutes ● Servings: 2

Calories 217 ● Calories from Fat 85 ● Total Fat 9.4 g ● Saturated Fat 1.3 g ● Monounsaturated Fat 6.6 g ● Cholesterol 0 mg ● Sodium 11 mg ● Carbohydrate 29.9 g ● Dietary Fiber 5.3 g ● Sugars 1.3 g ● Protein 3.1g

Exchanges: 2 starch, 1 1/2 fat

HELPFUL HINTS:

■ Any type of white-flesh fish, such as tilapia, flounder, or snapper, can be used as an alternative.

■ Any type of canned potatoes can be used. Be sure to rinse and drain the potatoes.

SHOPPING LIST

Seafood
3/4 pound sole fillets or other white-flesh fish

Dairy
1 small piece Parmesan cheese

Grocery
1 large can baby potatoes (1 pound needed) ⚡
1 jar dried dill
1 jar dried oregano

Produce
1 medium tomato

Staples
Olive oil
Olive oil spray
Salt
Black peppercorns

⚡ **SHOP SMART!**

Canned potatoes (per pound; 2 3/4 cups): 273 calories, 0.9 g fat, 59.8 g carbohydrate, 22 mg sodium

FISH IN A POUCH WITH GARLIC COUSCOUS

This is a wonderful way to cook fish. Sealed in a package with mushrooms and tomatoes, the fish steams in its own juices. Quick-cooking whole-wheat couscous takes only 5 minutes to make and has a nutty flavor.

Fish in a Pouch

1 cup sliced baby bello mushrooms (about 3 ounces)
2 6-ounce flounder fillets (or other thin fish fillet)
Salt and freshly ground black pepper

1/4 cup drained, sliced sun-dried tomatoes packed in olive oil (about 1 1/2 ounces) 🖈
1/4 cup fat-free low-sodium chicken broth

COUNTDOWN

- Preheat broiler.
- Start fish.
- While fish broils, make couscous.

1. Preheat broiler, and line a baking tray with foil. Cut two 10-inch-square pieces of foil.
2. Divide mushrooms between the foil pieces.
3. Place 1 fillet over the mushrooms. Sprinkle fish with salt and pepper to taste, and add the sun-dried tomato over top (if whole, cut into pieces with scissors).
4. Spoon chicken broth on top. Fold edges of foil together. Make sure they are tightly sealed.
5. Place on baking tray 5 inches from heat. Broil 15 minutes. Transfer to two dinner plates, and open foil just before serving.

Preparation time: 20 minutes ● Servings: 2

Calories 195 ● Calories from Fat 37 ● Total Fat 4.1 g ● Saturated Fat 0.8 g ● Monounsaturated 1.6 Fat g ● Cholesterol 84 mg ● Sodium 248 mg ● Carbohydrate 4.5 g ● Dietary Fiber 1.2 g ● Sugars 0 g ● Protein 34.2 g

Exchanges: 4 lean meat, 1 vegetable

Garlic Couscous

1 1/2 cups water
2/3 cup whole-wheat couscous
2 tablespoons olive oil
1 teaspoon minced garlic
Salt and freshly ground black pepper

1. Bring water to a boil over high heat. Stir in couscous.

2. Remove from heat, and cover with a lid. Let stand 5 minutes.

3. Remove lid, fluff with a fork, and add olive oil, garlic, and salt and pepper to taste. Toss well. Serve with fish.

Preparation time: 10 minutes ● Servings: 2

Calories 334 ● Calories from Fat 131 ● Total Fat 14.5 g ● Saturated Fat 1.9 g ● Monounsaturated Fat 9.8 g ● Cholesterol 0 mg ● Sodium 6 mg ● Carbohydrate 48.0 g ● Dietary Fiber 5.1 g ● Sugars 1.0 g ● Protein 8.2 g

Exchanges: 3 starch, 2 1/2 fat

HELPFUL HINTS:

■ Any type of fish fillet can be used, such as snapper, sole, or tilapia.

■ Any type of sliced mushrooms can be used.

■ Look for sliced sun-dried tomatoes. Packaged dehydrated sun-dried tomatoes can be used. Reconstitute them in hot water.

■ Minced garlic can be found in jars in the produce or condiment sections of the supermarket.

SHOPPING LIST

Seafood
2 6-ounce flounder fillets

Grocery
1 bottle sun-dried tomatoes packed in olive oil **!**
1 package whole-wheat couscous

Produce
3 ounces sliced baby bello mushrooms

Staples
Olive oil
Minced garlic
Fat-free, low-sodium chicken broth
Salt
Black peppercorns

! SHOP SMART!

Sun-dried tomatoes in olive oil (per 2 teaspoons): 21 calories, 1.4 g fat, 2.3 g carbohydrate, 27 mg sodium

GINGER-TERIYAKI STEAMED FISH AND CHINESE NOODLES

Ginger, teriyaki sauce, and scallions flavor this one-pot Asian steamed-fish meal. Chinese food takes only minutes to cook, but the chopping and cutting to prepare ingredients can be time-consuming. This recipe has very little preparation time and few ingredients, making it a very speedy Chinese supper.

Bok choy is a Chinese cabbage with white, thick stalks and dark green leaves. It's available year-round in the supermarket. Any type of firm lettuce, such as romaine, can be used.

Ginger-Teriyaki Steamed Fish and Chinese Noodles

3 tablespoons reduced-sodium teriyaki sauce ⚡
6 scallions, sliced (about 1 cup)
1 tablespoon chopped fresh ginger or
   1/2 teaspoon ground ginger
2 tablespoons sesame oil

3/4 pound flounder fillet
1 small head bok choy (about 2 cups leaves and 2 cups
   sliced stems)
1/4 pound steamed or fresh Chinese noodles

COUNTDOWN

■ Mix sauce and marinate snapper.
■ Place water in the bottom of a steamer and bring to a boil.
■ Prepare ingredients and steam.

1. Mix teriyaki sauce, scallions, ginger, and oil together in a bowl or self-sealing plastic bag. Add the flounder, and marinate 5 minutes, turning the fish over once during that time. Place water in steamer bottom, and bring to a boil.

2. Line the base of steamer basket with foil, and poke holes in the foil. Then line the basket with bok choy leaves, including the thick sliced stems. Spread noodles over bok choy.

3. Place fish on leaves, and pour marinade over top.

4. Cover with a lid, and steam 5 minutes over boiling water. Serve on two plates.

Preparation time: 15 minutes ● Servings: 2

Calories 477 ● Calories from Fat 159 ● Total Fat 17.6 g ● Saturated Fat 2.8 g ● Monounsaturated Fat 5.8 g ● Cholesterol 120 mg ● Sodium 625 mg ● Carbohydrate 37.6 g ● Dietary Fiber 3.8 g ● Sugars 5.3 g ● Protein 41.7 g

Exchanges: 2 starch, 1 vegetable, 5 lean meat, 1 1/2 fat

Here are some hints on alternatives to use for steaming equipment:

- Use a one- or two-tiered steamer. This is a large pot with one or two steaming inserts.
- Use a collapsible vegetable steaming rack placed in a skillet and covered with lid.
- Use a roasting pan with rack or broiler pan. Line rack with foil. Poke holes in the foil and place in roasting pan or in a large skillet. Cover tightly with foil (if you do not have a lid for the pan).
- Place a rack or perforated foil pie plate in a wok or other pan and cover with a lid.

HELPFUL HINTS:

- Any type of thin white fish fillet, such as tilapia, snapper, or sole, can be used as an alternative.
- Steamed or fresh Chinese noodles can be found in the produce section of the supermarket.
- Fresh angel hair pasta can be used instead of Chinese noodles.
- A quick way to slice scallions is to cut them with scissors.
- To help remove fish from steamer, line it with foil and poke holes in the foil. You can easily lift the foil out when the fish is cooked.

SHOPPING LIST

Seafood
3/4 pound flounder fillet

Grocery
1 bottle reduced-sodium teriyaki sauce ⚠
1 bottle sesame oil

Produce
1 bunch scallions
1 piece fresh ginger or ground ginger
1 small head bok choy
1 package steamed or fresh Chinese noodles

⚠ **SHOP SMART!**

Low-sodium teriyaki sauce (per tablespoon): 8 calories, 1.5 g carbohydrate, 168 mg sodium

CAJUN-BRONZED MAHI-MAHI WITH RICE AND SPINACH PILAF

This bronzed mahi-mahi is an alternative to blackened fish. It can cook indoors without smoke, and this method of cooking keeps the fish moist. The secret is to keep the skillet at the right temperature. The fish should take 7–8 minutes to cook. If it takes much longer, the skillet is not hot enough.

Using the Cajun spice mixture given in the recipe cuts down on the amount of salt found in prepared Cajun seasoning mixes.

A pilaf is a rice dish that originated in the Middle East. The rice is first sautéed in a skillet and then the liquid is added.

Cajun-Bronzed Mahi-Mahi

1/4 teaspoon cayenne pepper
1/2 teaspoon garlic powder
1 teaspoon dried oregano

1 teaspoon dried thyme
3/4 pound mahi-mahi fillet
1 tablespoon olive oil

COUNTDOWN

- Start rice.
- Mix spices.
- Make fish.
- Finish rice.

1. Mix cayenne pepper, garlic powder, oregano, and thyme together.
2. Spoon half of spice mixture onto one side of the fish, pressing it into the flesh.
3. Heat a skillet over high heat, and add the oil. When it is very hot, add the mahi-mahi, seasoned side down. Spread remaining spice mixture over top of the fish. Cook until the underside is bronze in color, 3–4 minutes.
4. Cook second side for 3–4 minutes or until cooked through. The fish is ready when a knife inserted into the flesh shows opaque rather than translucent meat. Serve.

Preparation time: 10 minutes ● Servings: 2

Calories 211 ● Calories from Fat 73 ● Total Fat 8.1 g ● Saturated Fat 1.4 g ● Monounsaturated Fat 5.1 g ● Cholesterol 126 mg ● Sodium 151 mg ● Carbohydrate 1.5 g ● Dietary Fiber 0.6 g ● Sugars 0 g ● Protein 31.7 g

Exchanges: 5 lean meat

Rice and Spinach Pilaf

2 teaspoons olive oil
1/2 cup long-grain white rice
1 cup low-sodium tomato juice ⚠️
1 cup water
3 cups washed ready-to-eat spinach

1. Heat olive oil in a medium nonstick skillet over medium-high heat.

2. Add rice, and sauté 1 minute. Add tomato juice and water.

3. Bring to a simmer, lower heat, cover, and gently simmer 15 minutes. If pan becomes dry, add a little more water.

4. Remove from heat, and stir in the spinach. Toss until it wilts in the heat of the rice. Serve.

Preparation time: 20 minutes ● Servings: 2

Calories 240 ● Calories from Fat 45 ● Total Fat 5.1 g ● Saturated Fat 0.7 g ● Monounsaturated Fat 3.4 g ● Cholesterol 0 mg ● Sodium 50 mg ● Carbohydrate 43.8 g ● Dietary Fiber 2.2 g ● Sugars 4.6g ● Protein 5.5 g

Exchanges: 2 1/2 starch, 1 vegetable, 1/2 fat

HELPFUL HINTS:

■ Any type of firm fish, such as grouper, farmed tilapia, or catfish, can be used.

SHOPPING LIST

Seafood
3/4 pound mahi-mahi fillet

Grocery
1 small bottle cayenne pepper
1 bottle garlic powder
1 bottle dried oregano
1 bottle dried thyme
1 package long-grain white rice
1 small bottle/can low-sodium
   tomato juice ⚠️

Produce
1 bag washed ready-to-eat spinach

Staples
Olive oil

⚠️ **SHOP SMART!**

Low-sodium tomato juice (per cup; 8 ounces): 41 calories, 10.3 g carbohydrate, 24 mg sodium

HALIBUT IN CIDER WITH SAFFRON RICE

This dish is from the Asturias region of northern Spain, located on the northern coast of the Iberian Peninsula, which is famous for its hard cider.

Hard cider is usually available in the autumn in many supermarkets. Apple juice can be used instead.

Halibut in Cider

3 tablespoons flour
3/4 pound halibut
2 teaspoons olive oil
Salt and freshly ground black pepper
2 teaspoons minced garlic

2 medium tomatoes, cut into 1/2-inch pieces
  (about 2 cups)
1 cup hard cider
2 tablespoons chopped fresh parsley

COUNTDOWN

■ Start rice.
■ Make halibut.
■ Complete rice.

1. Place flour on a plate and roll halibut in the flour, making sure all sides are coated.
2. Heat olive oil in a medium nonstick skillet over medium-high heat. Add halibut. Brown for 2 minutes; turn and brown second side 2 minutes. Transfer to a plate. Add salt and pepper to taste.
3. Add garlic, tomatoes, and cider to the skillet. Simmer 5 minutes.
4. Return fish to skillet, and cook in sauce 4 minutes.
5. To serve, spoon Saffron Rice onto a dinner plate and place halibut on top. Spoon sauce over fish, and sprinkle with parsley.

Preparation time: 20 minutes ● Servings: 2

Calories 360 ● Calories from Fat 81 ● Total Fat 9.0 g ● Saturated Fat 1.3 g ● Monounsaturated Fat 4.6 g ● Cholesterol 54 mg ● Sodium 108 mg ● Carbohydrate 23.2 g ● Dietary Fiber 2.8 g ● Sugars 4.9 g ● Protein 38.7 g

Exchanges: 1 1/2 carbohydrate, 5 lean meat, 1/2 fat

Saffron Rice

1 teaspoon olive oil
1 cup 10-minute brown rice (to make 1 1/2 cups cooked rice)
2 cups water
1/8 teaspoon saffron
Salt and freshly ground black pepper

1. Heat olive oil in a medium nonstick skillet over medium heat. Add rice, and toss 1 minute. Add water and saffron. Bring to a simmer. Cover. Simmer 10 minutes.
2. Add salt and pepper to taste. Serve with halibut.

Preparation time: 12 minutes ● Servings: 2

Calories 170 ● Calories from Fat 34 ● Total Fat 3.8 g ● Saturated Fat 0.6 g ● Monounsaturated Fat 2.1 g ● Cholesterol 0 mg ● Sodium 10 mg ● Carbohydrate 34.0 g ● Dietary Fiber 2.0 g ● Sugars 0 g ● Protein 3.0 g

Exchanges: 2 starch, 1/2 fat

HELPFUL HINTS:

■ Bijol or turmeric can be used instead of saffron for the rice.

■ Minced garlic can be found in jars in the produce or condiment sections of the supermarket.

■ A quick way to chop parsley is to wash, dry, and snip the leaves off the stem with scissors.

SHOPPING LIST

Seafood
3/4 pound halibut

Grocery
1 bottle hard cider or apple juice
1 box 10-minute brown rice
1 small package saffron

Produce
2 medium tomatoes
1 small bunch parsley

Staples
Flour
Olive oil
Minced garlic
Salt
Black peppercorns

FIVE-SPICE FILLET WITH CHINESE NOODLES AND SPROUTS

The pungent Chinese five-spice powder in this recipe gives the fish an intriguing flavor. Chinese five-spice powder is used in many Asian dishes and includes cinnamon, cloves, fennel seed, star anise, and Szechwan peppercorns. Use it to flavor meat, vegetables, rice, or noodles.

Preparing the ingredients for a Chinese dinner tends to take a little more time. But it's worth the effort when you're in the mood for Chinese food. These recipes provide the flavor without the sugar and salt normally found in Chinese dishes.

Five-Spice Fish Fillets

2 tablespoons flour
Salt and freshly ground black pepper
3/4 pound tilapia fillet
1/2 cup water

1 teaspoon Chinese five-spice powder
2 teaspoons minced garlic
1 tablespoon reduced-sodium soy sauce
3 teaspoons sesame oil, divided

COUNTDOWN

■ Place water for noodles on to boil.
■ Prepare ingredients.
■ Make fish.
■ Complete noodle dish.

1. Place flour on a plate, and season with salt and pepper to taste. Roll fish in flour.
2. Mix water, Chinese five-spice powder, garlic, soy sauce, and 2 teaspoons sesame oil together.
3. Heat remaining 1 teaspoon sesame oil over high heat in a medium skillet. Brown fish 2 minutes; turn and brown second side 2 minutes. Lower heat to medium, and add sauce. Simmer gently for 5 minutes, turning fish once.
4. Transfer fish to a plate, and spoon sauce over top.

Preparation time: 15 minutes ● Servings: 2

Calories 274 ● Calories from Fat 93 ● Total Fat 10.4 g ● Saturated Fat 2.3 g ● Monounsaturated Fat 4.2 g ● Cholesterol 84 mg ● Sodium 359 mg ● Carbohydrate 10.3 g ● Dietary Fiber 1.0 g ● Sugars 0.2 g ● Protein 36.4 g

Exchanges: 1/2 starch, 5 lean meat, 1/2 fat

Chinese Noodles and Sprouts

1/4 pound fresh or steamed Chinese noodles
1 cup fresh bean sprouts
3 scallions, sliced (1/2 cup)
2 teaspoons sesame oil
Salt and freshly ground black pepper

1. Bring a large pot with 2–3 quarts of water to a boil. Add Chinese noodles, and boil 3 minutes.

2. Add the bean sprouts; stir and drain into a colander. Return to saucepan.

3. Mix in scallions, oil, and salt and pepper to taste. Serve with the fish.

Preparation time: 5 minutes ● Servings: 2

Calories 209 ● Calories from Fat 56 ● Total Fat 6.3 g ● Saturated Fat 1.0 g ● Monounsaturated Fat 1.8 g ● Cholesterol 36 mg ● Sodium 15 mg ● Carbohydrate 31.9 g ● Dietary Fiber 2.6 g ● Sugars 3.8 g ● Protein 7.3 g

Exchanges: 2 starch, 1 fat

HELPFUL HINTS:

■ Chinese five-spice powder can be found in the spice section of the supermarket.

■ Minced garlic can be found in jars in the produce or condiment sections of the supermarket.

■ Any type of white fish fillet, such as snapper, sole, or grouper, can be used.

■ Dried Chinese noodles or angel hair pasta can be used. Cook according to package instructions.

■ A quick way to slice scallions is to snip them with scissors.

SOUTHWESTERN FISH FILLET WITH CHIPOTLE CORN AND ZUCCHINI

The spice section of the market will help you create this simple meal packed with punch. Prepackaged chili seasoning mix gives zip to the mild flavor and firm texture of farm-raised tilapia. Hot chipotle pepper powder from the spice section creates a sweet heat for the corn and zucchini.

Southwestern Fish Fillet

Olive oil spray
3/4 pound farm-raised tilapia
1 medium clove garlic, cut in half

2 teaspoons chili seasoning mix
2 teaspoons olive oil

COUNTDOWN

■ Preheat broiler.
■ Prepare ingredients.
■ Broil fish.
■ While fish cooks, prepare corn and zucchini.

1. Preheat broiler. Cover a baking tray with foil, and spray with olive oil spray.

2. Rinse tilapia and pat dry. Place on tray, rub one side of each fish fillet with the cut side of the garlic, and sprinkle evenly with chili seasoning mix.

3. Spoon olive oil over the fish.

4. Broil 6 inches from heat source until cooked through, 8 minutes. To test the tilapia, make a small cut into the thickest part. The flesh will be opaque, not translucent. Serve.

Preparation time: 12 minutes ● Servings: 2

Calories 233 ● Calories from Fat 90 ● Total Fat 10.0 g ● Saturated Fat 2.3 g ● Monounsaturated Fat 6.0 g ● Cholesterol 84mg ● Sodium 120 mg ● Carbohydrate 2.5 g ● Dietary Fiber 1.0 g ● Sugars 0.2 g ● Protein 34.6 g

Exchanges: 5 lean meat, 1/2 fat

Chipotle Corn and Zucchini

2 teaspoons olive oil
1/2 pound zucchini, cut into 1/2-inch pieces (about 1 3/4 cups)
2 cups frozen corn kernels
Large pinch chipotle chili pepper seasoning (about 1/8 teaspoon)
Salt

1. Heat oil in a nonstick skillet over medium-high heat.
2. Add the zucchini and corn. Sauté 5 minutes. Sprinkle with chipotle seasoning and salt to taste. Serve.

Preparation time: 8 minutes ● Servings: 2

Calories 187 ● Calories from Fat 61 ● Total Fat 6.8 g ● Saturated Fat 1.1 g
● Monounsaturated Fat 3.9 g ● Cholesterol 0 mg ● Sodium 45 mg ●
Carbohydrate 31.5 g ● Dietary Fiber 4.3 g ● Sugars 11.3 g ● Protein 6.3 g

Exchanges: 1 1/2 starch, 1 vegetable, 1 fat

HELPFUL HINTS:

■ If chipotle pepper seasoning is not available, use smoked or Hungarian paprika.

SHOPPING LIST

Seafood
3/4 pound farm-raised tilapia

Grocery
1 package chili seasoning mix
1 jar chipotle chili pepper seasoning
1 package frozen corn kernels

Produce
1/2 pound zucchini

Staples
Olive oil
Olive oil spray
Garlic
Salt

PECAN-CRUSTED TILAPIA WITH HOT PEPPER SUCCOTASH

Pecans and cornmeal create a crisp crust on these fresh tilapia fillets. Hot pepper jelly is a quick way to add flavor to vegetables. Here it spices up a traditional succotash for the side dish.

A general rule for cooking fish is to cook it for 10 minutes per inch of thickness, measured at the thickest part of the fish. I prefer to cook the fish 8 minutes. It will continue to cook when removed from the heat. To test for doneness, stick the point of a knife into the thickest section and gently pull some of the meat away. The flesh should be opaque, but juicy. The fish will continue to cook in its own heat after it is removed from the stove.

Pecan-Crusted Tilapia

3 tablespoons chopped, unsalted pecans

1 tablespoon coarse cornmeal

1 egg white

3/4 pound tilapia fillet

1 tablespoon olive oil

Salt and freshly ground black pepper

COUNTDOWN

■ Prepare the ingredients.
■ Make the succotash.
■ Make the snapper.

1. Place pecans and cornmeal on a plate.

2. Lightly beat the egg white. Dip the tilapia into the egg white and then into the chopped pecans, making sure all sides are covered. Gently press pecans into the flesh.

3. Heat the oil in a nonstick skillet over medium-high heat. Add the tilapia, and sauté 4 minutes; turn and sauté another 4 minutes. To test for doneness, stick the point of a knife into the thickest section and gently pull some of the meat away. The flesh should be opaque, but juicy. Cook a minute longer, if necessary.

4. Sprinkle with salt and pepper to taste and serve.

Preparation time: 15 minutes ● Servings: 2

Calories 312 ● Calories from Fat 148 ● Total Fat 16.4 g ● Saturated Fat 2.8 g ● Monounsaturated Fat 9.8 g ● Cholesterol 84 mg ● Sodium 118 mg ● Carbohydrate 5.3 g ● Dietary Fiber 1.1 g ● Sugars 0.6 g ● Protein 37.2 g

Exchanges: 1/2 carbohydrate, 5 lean meat, 1 1/2 fat

Hot Pepper Succotash

1 cup frozen corn kernels
1 cup frozen lima beans
2 tablespoons hot pepper jelly

Microwave method
Place all ingredients in a microwave-safe bowl. Cover. Microwave on high 2 minutes. Toss well. Makes 2 servings. Serve.

Stove-top method
Place all ingredients in a skillet over medium-high heat. Sauté 3 minutes. The vegetables only need to be warmed through. Serve.

Preparation time: 5 minutes ● Servings: 2

Calories 221 ● Calories from Fat 12 ● Total Fat 1.3 g ● Saturated Fat 0.3 g ● Monounsaturated Fat 0.3 g ● Cholesterol 0 mg ● Sodium 57 mg ● Carbohydrate 46.9 g ● Dietary Fiber 6.4 g ● Sugars 4.5 g ● Protein 8.6 g

Exchanges: 2 starch, 1 carbohydrate

HELPFUL HINTS:

■ Any type of fish fillet can be used.

■ Chop the pecans in a food processor.

SHOPPING LIST

Seafood
3/4 pound tilapia fillet

Grocery
1 small package unsalted pecans
1 package coarse cornmeal
1 jar hot pepper jelly
1 package frozen corn kernels
1 package frozen lima beans

Staples
Olive oil
Egg
Salt
Black peppercorns

FISH CHOWDER WITH GREEN SALAD

The essence of this dish is the sweet flavor of fresh fish. Select whatever fish looks best that day. Try to choose a fairly firm fish, such as tilapia. There is no flour in this chowder, making it very light and allowing the fresh ingredients to stand out.

Fish Chowder

Olive oil spray
2 ounces smoked lean ham, cut into strips
   (about 1/2 cup) 🔲
2 cups fresh diced onion
1 cup fresh diced celery
1 pound canned potatoes, rinsed and drained
   (about 2 1/2 cups)
1 cup low-sodium V8 juice 🔲

1 cup water
3/4 pound tilapia or mahi-mahi
1/2 tablespoon dried thyme
1 teaspoon dried tarragon
2 tablespoons half and half
1 teaspoon olive oil
Salt and freshly ground black pepper

COUNTDOWN

◼ Make chowder.
◼ Make salad.

1. Heat a medium saucepan over medium-high heat, and spray with olive oil spray. Add ham, onion, and celery. Sauté 3 minutes, stirring occasionally.

2. Cut potatoes in half, and add to saucepan with V8 juice and water. Cover with a lid, and simmer 3 minutes.

3. While potatoes cook, rinse fish, pat dry, and cut into 2-inch pieces. Reduce heat to medium, and add fish, thyme, and tarragon. Simmer (do not boil) covered, 3 minutes. Remove from heat, and add half and half, olive oil, and salt and pepper to taste. Serve.

Preparation time: 12 minutes ● Servings: 2

Calories 486 ● Calories from Fat 95 ● Total Fat 10.6 g ● Saturated Fat 3.4 g ● Monounsaturated Fat 5.1 g ● Cholesterol 103 mg ● Sodium 470 mg ● Carbohydrate 53.8 g ● Dietary Fiber 9.7 g ● Sugars 13.3 g ● Protein 46.3 g

Exchanges: 2 1/2 starch, 2 vegetable, 5 lean meat, 1/2 fat

Green Salad

4 cups washed ready-to-eat salad
2 tablespoons reduced-fat vinaigrette dressing 🔼

1. Add salad to a bowl. Toss with salad dressing. Serve.

Preparation time: 3 minutes ● Servings: 2

Calories 27 ● Calories from Fat 11 ● Total Fat 1.2 g ● Saturated Fat 0.1 g ● Monounsaturated Fat 0.3 g ● Cholesterol 1 mg ● Sodium 12 mg ● Carbohydrate 3.8 g ● Dietary Fiber 2.0 g ● Sugars 1.8 g ● Protein 1.2 g

Exchanges: 1 vegetable

HELPFUL HINTS:

■ Low-sodium tomato juice can be used.

■ Diced fresh onions and celery can be found in the produce section of the supermarket.

SHOPPING LIST

Seafood
3/4 pound tilapia or mahi-mahi

Deli
2 ounces smoked, lean ham 🔼

Dairy
1 carton half and half

Grocery
1 can whole potatoes
1 8-ounce can low-sodium V8 juice 🔼
1 bottle dried thyme
1 bottle dried tarragon

Produce
1 container fresh diced onion (2 cups needed)
1 container diced celery
1 bag washed ready-to-eat salad

Staples
Olive oil spray
Olive oil
Reduced-fat vinaigrette dressing 🔼
Salt
Black peppercorns

🔼 SHOP SMART!

Lean ham (per ounce): 30 calories, 0.7 g fat, 0.2 g saturated fat, 301 mg sodium

Low-sodium V8 juice (per cup; 8 ounces): 51 calories, 10.0 g carbohydrate, 141 mg sodium

Reduced-fat vinaigrette or oil and vinegar dressing (per tablespoon): 11 calories, 1.0 g fat, 4 mg sodium

MEXICAN ORANGE FILLET WITH FRIED CORN AND GREEN PEPPER

Sautéing a fish fillet in a savory orange sauce makes for an unusual, tangy Mexican dish. Fried corn tossed with green peppers completes this meal. Until recently, most food lovers thought of Mexican cooking in terms of tacos, tamales, and tongue-scorching salsas, but more people are beginning to savor the subtle flavor distinctions that make Mexican food a truly great cuisine.

Mexican Orange Fillet

2 tablespoons flour
3/4 pound fish fillets (white, non-oily fish, such as tilapia, sole, or flounder)
1 teaspoon canola oil

1/2 cup frozen diced onion
1 teaspoon minced garlic
Salt and freshly ground black pepper
1 cup orange juice

COUNTDOWN

■ Make corn, and transfer to two dinner plates.
■ Using same skillet, make fish.

1. Place flour on a plate.
2. Rinse fish fillet and pat dry with a paper towel. Dip into flour, making sure both sides are coated.
3. Heat oil in the skillet used for the corn over medium-high heat. Add the fish. Brown fish 2 minutes; turn and brown 2 minutes. Add onion and garlic. Transfer fish to a plate, and add salt and pepper to taste.
4. Stir orange juice into the skillet, scraping up the brown bits in the bottom.
5. Lower heat to medium, and return fish to skillet. Cover with a lid and cook, gently, 2–3 minutes for fish that is 3/4-inch thick. Cook 5 minutes for 1-inch thick fish. Remove from skillet and serve.

Preparation time: 15 minutes ● Servings: 2

Calories 285 ● Calories from Fat 51 ● Total Fat 5.6 g ● Saturated Fat 1.5 g ● Monounsaturated Fat 2.6 g ● Cholesterol 84 mg ● Sodium 94 mg ● Carbohydrate 23.2 g ● Dietary Fiber 1.2 g ● Sugars 1.8 g ● Protein 36.6 g

Exchanges: 1 1/2 carbohydrate, 5 lean meat

Fried Sweet Corn (Esquites)

1 tablespoon canola oil
1 cup frozen, diced onion
1 cup frozen, diced green bell pepper
1 cup frozen corn kernels
Several drops hot pepper sauce
Salt
10 baked tortilla chips, broken into halves (or quarters, if large)

1. Heat oil in a nonstick skillet over medium-high heat. Add the onion, green bell pepper, and corn. Sauté 5 minutes.
2. Sprinkle with hot pepper sauce and salt to taste. Spoon onto dinner plates, and top with tortilla chips.

Preparation time: 7 minutes ● Servings: 2

Calories 207 ● Calories from Fat 82 ● Total Fat 9.1 g ● Saturated Fat 1.0 g ● Monounsaturated Fat 5.1 g ● Cholesterol 0 mg ● Sodium 103 mg ● Carbohydrate 30.3 g ● Dietary Fiber 4.5 g ● Sugars 9.8 g ● Protein 4.6 g

Exchanges: 1 1/2 starch, 1 vegetable, 1 1/2 fat

HELPFUL HINTS:

■ Any type of non-oily fish fillet can be used. Timing is for a fish that is 1-inch thick. Add a few more minutes for a thicker piece.

■ Minced garlic can be found in jars in the produce or condiment sections of the supermarket.

■ Frozen onion is used in both recipes. Measure for both at the same time.

■ Use the same skillet for the Fried Corn and Fish.

SHOPPING LIST

Seafood
3/4 pound fish fillets (white, non-oily fish, such as tilapia, sole, or flounder)

Grocery
1 bottle hot pepper sauce
1 small package baked tortilla chips
1 small carton orange juice
1 package frozen corn kernels
1 package frozen diced green bell pepper
1 package frozen diced onion

Produce
1 green bell pepper

Staples
Flour
Canola oil
Minced garlic
Salt
Black peppercorns

SAUTÉED FISH WITH PINEAPPLE SALSA AND POBLANO RICE

It's easy to see why salsa is one of America's favorite condiments. Its fresh, crisp, tangy flavor adds a refreshing touch to a meal without adding a lot of sugar or fat. This bright pineapple salsa brings out the flavor of fresh fish.

The poblano peppers (called ancho peppers when dried) that give the rice dish its zing are medium-hot. Jalapeño peppers can be used instead. Use 2 tablespoons jalapeño peppers if you choose to substitute.

Sautéed Fish with Pineapple Salsa

1 cup fresh pineapple, coarsely chopped
3/4 cup tomato salsa *!*

1 tablespoon canola oil
3/4 pound fish fillets (such as tilapia)

COUNTDOWN

■ Start rice.
■ Make salsa.
■ Finish rice.
■ Cook fish.

1. Mix pineapple and tomato salsa together, and set aside.
2. Heat oil in a nonstick skillet over medium-high heat.
3. Add fish, and sauté 5 minutes. Turn and sauté 3 minutes, or according to size of fish. Fish is done when it is opaque and not translucent.
4. Place on two dinner plates, and serve some of the salsa on top and the rest on the side.

Preparation time: 12 minutes ● Servings: 2

Calories 290 ● Calories from Fat 91 ● Total Fat 10.1 g ● Saturated Fat 1.9 g ● Monounsaturated Fat 5.4 g ● Cholesterol 84 mg ● Sodium 286 mg ● Carbohydrate 15.7 g ● Dietary Fiber2.5 g ● Sugars 3.0 g ● Protein 36 g

Exchanges: 1/2 fruit, 1 vegetable, 5 lean meat, 1/2 fat

Poblano Rice

1 package microwave brown rice (1 1/2 cups cooked)
2 tablespoons seeded, chopped poblano pepper
2 teaspoons canola oil

1. Microwave rice according to package instructions. Measure 1 1/2 cup rice, and reserve remaining rice for another time. Add the poblano pepper and oil. Toss well. Serve.

Preparation time: 5 minutes ● Servings: 2

Calories 222 ● Calories from Fat 64 ● Total Fat 7.1 g ● Saturated Fat 0.7 g ● Monounsaturated Fat 3.6 g ● Cholesterol 0 mg ● Sodium 12 mg ● Carbohydrate 29.8 g ● Dietary Fiber 1.5 g ● Sugars 0 g ● Protein 3.9 g

Exchanges: 2 starch, 1 1/2 fat

HELPFUL HINTS:

■ Any fresh non-oily fish fillet can be used. For cooking the fish fillet, plan on 10 minutes per inch of thickness.

■ Look for fresh pineapple cubes in the produce section. Chop them in the food processor.

SHOPPING LIST

Seafood
3/4 pound fish fillets (such as tilapia)

Grocery
1 jar tomato salsa *!*
1 package microwave brown rice

Produce
1 container fresh pineapple cubes
1 small poblano pepper

Staples
Canola oil

! SHOP SMART!

Salsa (per 2 tablespoons):
10 calories, 2 g carbohydrate, 65 mg sodium
[*Example*: Newman's Own All-Natural Bandito Salsa]

BRAISED CHINESE SHRIMP

This is a quick one-pot meal. The total cooking time for this dinner is just 7 minutes. Add 10 minutes to the preparation time and the meal can be ready in less than 20 minutes.

For easy stir-frying, place all of the prepared ingredients on a cutting board or plate in the order you'll be using them. You won't have to look at the recipe once you start to cook. Make sure your wok is very hot before adding the ingredients.

Braised Chinese Shrimp

1 tablespoon reduced-sodium soy sauce
2 tablespoons sherry
2 tablespoons honey
3/4 pound peeled shrimp
1 1/2 tablespoons sesame oil, divided
3 cups fresh sliced cabbage

2 cups fresh diced cucumber
2 teaspoons minced garlic
3 cups fresh bean sprouts
2 teaspoons ground ginger
4 scallions, sliced (about 2/3 cup)
2 tablespoons sliced almonds

COUNTDOWN

■ Prepare all ingredients.
■ Complete dish.

1. Mix the soy sauce, sherry, and honey together; add shrimp and set aside.

2. Heat 1/2 tablespoon sesame oil in a wok or skillet over high heat until smoking.

3. Add the cabbage, cucumber, garlic, bean sprouts, and ginger, and stir-fry 1 minute.

4. Remove shrimp from sauce, reserving sauce. Add to the work. Stir-fry 3 minutes, turning shrimp over once or twice. Shrimp will turn pink.

5. Spoon shrimp and vegetables onto a plate.

6. Add sauce to wok and boil to reduce by half, about 2–3 minutes. Pour sauce over shrimp and vegetables.

7. Sprinkle scallions on top, and the sliced almonds over the scallions. Serve.

Preparation time: 15 minutes ● Servings: 2

Calories 524 ● Calories from Fat 166 ● Total Fat 18.5 g ● Saturated Fat 2.5 g ● Monounsaturated Fat 7.5 g ● Cholesterol 258 mg ● Sodium 562 mg ● Carbohydrate 46.5 g ● Dietary Fiber 8.5 g ● Sugars 30.2 g ● Protein 44.9 g

Exchanges: 1 carbohydrate, 5 vegetable, 5 lean meat, 2 fat

HELPFUL HINTS:

- Buy peeled shrimp.

- Shredded or sliced cabbage can be found packaged in the produce section of most markets.

- Minced garlic can be found in jars in the produce or condiment sections of the supermarket.

- Fresh diced cucumber is available in the produce section of the supermarket.

SHOPPING LIST

Seafood
3/4 pound peeled shrimp

Grocery
1 bottle reduced-sodium soy sauce
1 small bottle sherry
1 bottle sesame oil
1 package sliced almonds
1 bottle ground ginger

Produce
1 package fresh sliced or shredded cabbage
1 container fresh diced cucumber
1 package fresh bean sprouts
1 bunch scallions

Staples
Honey
Minced garlic

SWEET AND SOUR SHRIMP WITH BROWN RICE

Using sliced onions and green pepper from the produce section of the market helps you make this dinner in just 5 minutes.

Sweet and Sour Shrimp

Olive oil spray
1 cup fresh diced onion
1 cup fresh diced green bell pepper

3/4 pound peeled shrimp
1 cup tomato wedges
1/3 cup low-sodium sweet and sour sauce 🔳

COUNTDOWN

■ Prepare ingredients.
■ Make rice, and spoon onto dinner plates.
■ Make shrimp.

1. Heat wok or skillet over high heat, and spray with olive oil spray.
2. When smoking, add onion and green bell pepper. Stir-fry 2 minutes.
3. Transfer vegetables to bowl, and add shrimp and tomatoes to wok. Stir-fry 1 minute.
4. Add sweet and sour sauce to wok, and immediately return vegetables to wok. Toss 30 seconds. Serve over rice.

Preparation time: 5 minutes ● Servings: 2

Calories 304 ● Calories from Fat 43 ● Total Fat 4.8 g ● Saturated Fat 0.9 g ● Monounsaturated Fat 1.5 g ● Cholesterol 258 mg ● Sodium 517 mg ● Carbohydrate 28.4 g ● Dietary Fiber 3.7 g ● Sugars 16.9 g ● Protein 36.8 g

Exchanges: 1 carbohydrate, 2 vegetable, 4 lean meat

Brown Rice

1 package microwaveable brown rice (for 1 1/2 cups cooked rice)
1 tablespoon olive oil
Salt and freshly ground black pepper

1. Microwave rice according to package instructions. Measure 1 1/2 cups cooked rice into a bowl. Reserve the rest for another use.

2. Add olive oil and salt and pepper to taste. Toss well, and spoon onto two dinner plates. Serve shrimp on top.

Preparation time: 5 minutes ● Servings: 2

Calories 240 ● Calories from Fat 84 ● Total Fat 9.3 g ● Saturated Fat 1.3 g ● Monounsaturated Fat 5.7 g ● Cholesterol 0 mg ● Sodium 11 mg ● Carbohydrate 29.3 g ● Dietary Fiber 1.5 g ● Sugars 0 g ● Protein 3.8 g

Exchanges: 2 starch, 2 fat

HELPFUL HINTS:

■ Diced fresh onions and green bell peppers can be found in the produce section of the supermarket.

■ Make sure your wok or skillet is very hot. Add the food to the hot wok and don't touch it for about 30 seconds. This gives the wok a chance to regain its heat.

SHOPPING LIST

Seafood
3/4 pound peeled shrimp

Grocery
1 small bottle low-sodium sweet and sour sauce **!**
1 small package microwaveable brown rice

Produce
1 container fresh diced onion
1 container fresh diced green bell pepper
1 medium tomato

Staples
Olive oil
Olive oil spray
Salt
Black peppercorns

! **SHOP SMART!**

Low-sodium sweet and sour sauce (per tablespoon): 35 calories, 190 mg sodium
[*Example*: Kikkoman brand]

SPAGHETTI DEL PESCATORE (FISHERMAN'S SPAGHETTI) WITH CELERY AND FENNEL SALAD

Spaghetti del Pescatore (Fisherman's Spaghetti) is the kind of simple dish that makes Italian food so enticing. This dish has origins on the tiny island of Elba, off the western coast of Italy, and I adapted it to come up with this dish. This recipe uses mussels and shrimp, but any shellfish, including clams or lobster, may be substituted.

The accompanying salad uses fennel, a pale green bulb with darker, feathery leaves. It has a similar texture to celery and a very mild licorice flavor.

Spaghetti del Pescatore (Fisherman's Spaghetti)

1 pound fresh mussels
1 teaspoon minced garlic
1/8 teaspoon crushed red pepper
1/2 cup dry white wine
3/4 pound peeled and deveined shrimp

1 cup low-sodium, low-fat tomato sauce ⚡
1/2 cup chopped parsley
Salt and freshly ground black pepper
3 ounces spaghetti (1 rounded cup, cooked)
2 teaspoons olive oil

COUNTDOWN

■ Place water for pasta on to boil.
■ Make salad and let marinate.
■ Make spaghetti dish.

1. Place a large saucepan filled with water on to boil for pasta.
2. Scrub mussels and place in a medium nonstick skillet over medium-high heat. Cover with a lid, and cook until shells open, about 2 minutes, shaking pan several times. Transfer mussels to a bowl, leaving the juice in the pan. Discard any mussels that are not open. (If juice is sandy, strain through a sieve lined with paper towels.)
3. Add the garlic, crushed red pepper, and white wine to the skillet. Boil to reduce liquid for about 1 minute.
4. Lower heat to medium, and add shrimp and tomato sauce. Simmer, uncovered, 2 minutes or until shrimp are pink; remove from heat. Sprinkle with parsley, and add salt and pepper to taste.
5. Return mussels to skillet, remove skillet from heat, cover, and set aside.
6. Cook spaghetti in boiling water, 8–9 minutes. Drain and toss with olive oil and salt and pepper to taste. Serve on plate, and top with shrimp and mussel sauce.

Preparation time: 15 minutes ● Servings: 2

Calories 548 ● Calories from Fat 91 ● Total Fat 10.1 g ● Saturated Fat 0.7 g ● Monounsaturated Fat 4.2 g ● Cholesterol 278 mg ● Sodium 483 mg ● Carbohydrate 50.3 g ● Dietary Fiber 3.8 g ● Sugars 8.3 g ● Protein 50.8 g

Exchanges: 2 starch, 2 vegetable, 1/2 carbohydrate, 6 lean meat

Celery and Fennel Salad

2 celery stalks (about 1 cup sliced)
1 small fennel bulb (about 2 cups sliced)
2 tablespoons reduced-fat vinaigrette dressing ⚠
Salt and freshly ground black pepper

1. Remove leaves from celery and fennel. Chop some of the fennel leaves to make about 2 tablespoons chopped leaves.
2. Thinly slice, paper thin if possible, the celery and fennel. Place in a bowl, and add the dressing. Toss well. Sprinkle chopped fennel leaves on top, and add salt and pepper to taste. Serve.

Preparation time: 5 minutes ● Servings: 2

Calories 46 ● Calories from Fat 11 ● Total Fat 1.2 g ● Saturated Fat 0.1 g ● Monounsaturated Fat 0.4 g ● Cholesterol 1 mg ● Sodium 90 mg ● Carbohydrate 8.5 g ● Dietary Fiber 3.5 g ● Sugars 1.6 g ● Protein 1.5 g

Exchanges: 2 vegetable

HELPFUL HINTS:

■ Crushed red pepper can be found in the spice section of the supermarket.
■ Buy pre-shelled shrimp.
■ Wash mussels under cold water. Tap mussels that are open to see if they will close. Discard any that remain open.
■ Minced garlic can be found in the produce section of most markets.
■ Slice the celery and fennel in a food processor, using the thin slicing blade.
■ A quick way to chop fennel leaves is to snip them with scissors.

Short cut tip: Skip the Celery and Fennel Salad and use a washed ready-to-eat Italian-style salad instead.

SHOPPING LIST

Seafood
1 pound fresh mussels
3/4 pound peeled and deveined shrimp

Grocery
1 bottle crushed red pepper
1 bottle dry white wine
1 bottle/can low-sodium, low-fat tomato sauce ⚠
1 package spaghetti

Produce
1 bunch parsley
1 bunch celery
1 small fennel bulb

Staples
Olive oil
Minced garlic
Reduced-fat vinaigrette dressing ⚠
Salt
Black peppercorns

⚠ SHOP SMART!

Low-sodium tomato sauce (per cup; 8 ounces): 103 calories, 0.5 g fat, 21.3 g carbohydrate, 21 mg sodium

Reduced-fat vinaigrette or oil and vinegar dressing (per tablespoon): 11 calories, 1.0 g fat, 4 mg sodium

LEMON-PEPPER SHRIMP AND COUSCOUS ON A BED OF SPINACH

Hot and spicy, this tasty one-pot meal features lemon-pepper shrimp combined with couscous and olives and can be prepared in 15 minutes. The shrimp marinates for a few minutes in lemon juice and cracked black pepper while you prepare the remaining ingredients.

Lemon-Pepper Shrimp and Couscous on a Bed of Spinach

1 tablespoon olive oil
2 tablespoons lemon juice
1/2 tablespoon cracked black peppercorns
10 ounces peeled, cooked shrimp
1 cup fresh diced onion

1 1/2 teaspoons minced garlic
1/2 cup whole-wheat couscous
1 cup low-sodium V8 juice
8 pitted black olives
4 cups washed ready-to-eat spinach

COUNTDOWN

- Marinate the shrimp.
- Prepare the remaining ingredients.
- Complete the recipe.

1. Mix olive oil, lemon juice, and black pepper together in a bowl or self-sealing plastic bag. Add shrimp, and marinate for 5 minutes while the rest of the ingredients are prepared.
2. Remove shrimp from marinade, and set aside. Reserve marinade.
3. Heat a nonstick skillet over medium-high heat, and add marinade. Add onion, garlic, and couscous. Sauté 1 minute.
4. Add V8 juice to the skillet with the olives. Bring to a simmer, cover with a lid, and gently simmer for 5 minutes.
5. Add shrimp. Simmer, covered, for 2 minutes or until warm through.
6. Place spinach in a bowl, and microwave on high 1 minute. Divide spinach between two dinner plates. Spoon shrimp and couscous over spinach.

Preparation time: 20 minutes ● Servings: 2

Calories 502 ● Calories from Fat 110 ● Total Fat 12.2 g ● Saturated Fat 1.8 g ● Monounsaturated Fat 6.4 g ● Cholesterol 258 mg ● Sodium 490 mg ● Carbohydrate 56.2 g ● Dietary Fiber 8.3 g ● Sugars 4.8 g ● Protein 45 g

Exchanges: 2 1/2 starch, 3 vegetable, 4 lean meat, 1 fat

HELPFUL HINTS:

■ Diced fresh onions can be found in the produce section of the supermarket.

■ Frozen diced onion can be used instead of the fresh chopped onion.

■ Cracked black pepper can be found in the spice section of the market.

■ Minced garlic can be found in jars in the produce or condiment sections of the supermarket.

SHOPPING LIST

Seafood
10 ounces peeled, cooked shrimp

Grocery
1 bottle lemon juice
1 bottle cracked black peppercorns
1 package whole-wheat couscous
1 small bottle/can low-sodium V8 juice **!**
1 small can pitted black olives

Produce
1 bag washed ready-to-eat spinach
1 container fresh diced onion

Staples
Olive oil
Minced garlic

! SHOP SMART!

Low-sodium V8 juice (per cup; 8 ounces): 51 calories, 10.0 g carbohydrate, 141 mg sodium

SHRIMP AND POBLANO PEPPER TACOS WITH PINTO BEAN SALAD

You'll love these delicious tacos for the charred poblano peppers and shrimp and because they're simple to prepare. If you are pressed for time, skip charring the poblano peppers. The flavor will be different, but the taco will still be tasty.

Shrimp and Poblano Pepper Tacos

1/2 cup sliced poblano pepper
4 6-inch corn tortillas
2 teaspoons olive oil
1/2 cup frozen chopped onion

3/4 pound peeled and deveined shrimp
1 teaspoon bottled lemon juice
Salt and freshly ground black pepper
2 tablespoons chopped cilantro

COUNTDOWN

- Place peppers under boiler.
- Prepare the ingredients.
- Assemble the pinto bean salad.
- Make shrimp dish.

1. Preheat broiler. Place poblano peppers on a foil-lined tray and place under the broiler for 5 minutes to char the peppers. Broil until the skin turns black. Turn peppers, and char for 3 minutes.

2. While peppers char, wrap the tortillas in foil and place on a lower shelf in the oven to warm, about 5 minutes.

3. Remove tortillas, and keep warm in foil until ready to use. Remove the peppers, and cut into strips, removing seeds.

4. Heat the oil in a medium nonstick skillet over medium-high heat. Add the onion. Cook 2 minutes.

5. Add the shrimp, and cook 3 minutes, stirring several times.

6. Remove from heat. Toss with lemon juice and salt and pepper to taste. Sprinkle with chopped cilantro.

7. Divide the shrimp and pepper slices among the tortillas, and fold in half into a taco shape. Serve two tacos per person.

Preparation time: 15 minutes ● Servings: 2

Calories 362 ● Calories from Fat 80 ● Total Fat 8.8 g ● Saturated Fat 1.4 g ● Monounsaturated Fat 4.1 g ● Cholesterol 258 mg ● Sodium 261 mg ● Carbohydrate 31.9 g ● Dietary Fiber 3.5 g ● Sugars 2.2 g ● Protein 38.4 g

Exchanges: 2 starch, 5 lean meat

Pinto Bean Salad

2 tablespoons reduced-fat vinaigrette dressing ⚠
3/4 cup canned pinto beans, rinsed and drained
2 cups shredded lettuce
2 cups tomato wedges
2 tablespoons chopped cilantro
Salt and freshly ground black pepper

1. Place dressing in a medium bowl.
2. Add the beans, lettuce, and tomatoes. Toss well. Add cilantro and salt and pepper to taste. Serve.

Preparation time: 5 minutes ● Servings: 2

Calories 129 ● Calories from Fat 20 ● Total Fat 2.2 g ● Saturated Fat 0.3 g ● Monounsaturated Fat 0.5 g ● Cholesterol 1 mg ● Sodium 176 mg ● Carbohydrate 23.1g ● Dietary Fiber 7.4 g ● Sugars 6.0 g ● Protein 6.6 g

Exchanges: 1 starch, 1 vegetable, 1/2 fat

HELPFUL HINTS:

■ Cilantro is used in both recipes, prepare it all at one time and divide for the recipes.

SHOPPING LIST

Seafood
3/4 pound peeled and deveined shrimp

Grocery
1 package 6-inch corn tortillas
1 can pinto beans
1 package frozen chopped onion
1 bottle lemon juice

Produce
2 poblano peppers
1 bunch cilantro
1 package shredded lettuce
2 medium tomatoes

Staples
Olive oil
Reduced-fat vinaigrette dressing ⚠
Salt
Black peppercorns

⚠ **SHOP SMART!**

Reduced-fat vinaigrette or oil and vinegar dressing (per tablespoon): 11 calories, 1.0 g fat, 4 mg sodium

BLACK BEAN SOUP WITH SHRIMP

Adding shrimp to this hearty black bean soup turns it into a welcoming meal. Best of all, it takes only 20 minutes from start to finish. This is the type of meal you can make without a trip to the supermarket. Keep canned beans (any type can be used), frozen shrimp, canned tomatoes, and chicken broth on hand.

Black Bean Soup with Shrimp

1 tablespoon olive oil
3/4 pound peeled shrimp
1 cup fresh diced onion
2 teaspoons minced garlic
2 cups canned black beans, rinsed and drained
1 cup low-sodium canned diced tomatoes, drained **!**

1 cup fat-free, low-sodium chicken broth
1 cup water
1 teaspoon ground cumin
Salt and freshly ground black pepper
Several drops hot pepper sauce
2 tablespoons chopped cilantro (*optional*)

COUNTDOWN

■ Sauté shrimp.
■ Cook remaining ingredients.

1. Heat oil in a large saucepan over medium-high heat. Add shrimp, and sauté 2 minutes; turn after 1 minute or until shrimp turn pink. Transfer to a plate.

2. Add onion to pan, and sauté 1 minute.

3. Add the garlic, black beans, tomatoes, chicken broth, and water. Bring to a boil, and cook 10 minutes. Add cumin and salt and black pepper to taste.

4. Return shrimp to saucepan for a few seconds to warm through.

5. Add hot pepper sauce or place on the table for each person to add as they like. Serve in large soup bowls, and sprinkle cilantro on top (*optional*).

Preparation time: 20 minutes ● Servings: 2

Calories 530 ● Calories from Fat 100 ● Total Fat 11.2 g ● Saturated Fat 1.8 g ● Monounsaturated Fat 5.6 g ● Cholesterol 258 mg ● Sodium 566 mg ● Carbohydrate 55.5 g ● Dietary Fiber 17.5 g ● Sugars 5.4 g ● Protein 53.4 g

Exchanges: 3 starch, 1 vegetable, 6 lean meat

HELPFUL HINTS:

■ Any type of canned tomatoes can be used.

■ Diced fresh onions can be found in the produce section of the supermarket.

■ Minced garlic can be found in jars in the produce or condiment sections of the supermarket.

■ Hot pepper sauce is added at the end. The heat is up to you.

■ A quick way to chop cilantro is to snip the leaves with scissors.

SHRIMP MUSHROOM QUESADILLAS AND BLACK BEAN AND TOMATO SALAD

These quesadillas are little Tex-Mex sandwiches that are pan-fried and served with a quick Black Bean and Tomato Salad. The variety of textures and flavors—from the earthy, meaty mushrooms to the soft cheese and crisp tortillas—creates a tasty, satisfying meal.

The mushrooms and spinach are precooked, which can be done in the same skillet that will be used to cook the quesadillas or in a microwave oven.

Shrimp Mushroom Quesadillas

1/4 pound sliced, baby bello mushrooms (1 1/2 cups)
2 cups washed ready-to-eat spinach
Salt and freshly ground black pepper
Olive oil spray

4 6-inch corn tortillas
10 ounces cooked, medium, peeled shrimp
6 tablespoons shredded, reduced-fat Cheddar cheese (1 1/2 ounces) *l*

COUNTDOWN

■ Make side dish and set aside.
■ Make quesadilla.

Stove-top method

1. Heat a nonstick skillet over medium-high heat. Add the mushrooms, and sauté 2 minutes or until mushrooms are soft. Stir in spinach until it wilts, about 1 minute. Drain, transfer to a bowl, and add salt and pepper to taste.

Microwave method

1. Place mushrooms in a microwave-safe bowl, and microwave on high 2 minutes. Remove from microwave, stir in spinach, and return to the microwave on high for 1 minute. Stir to combine ingredients. Drain, and add salt and pepper to taste.

2. Heat two nonstick skillets over medium-high heat, and spray with olive oil spray.

3. Add 2 tortillas, and heat about 1 minute or until bottom is golden.

4. Turn over and spoon 1/4 of the mushrooms and spinach mixture over half of each of the tortillas.

5. Place 1/4 of the shrimp on top of each tortilla, and sprinkle 1 1/2 tablespoons of the shredded cheese over the shrimp on each tortilla.

6. Gently fold in half, cover with a lid, and sauté 1 minute. Turn over, cover, and sauté 1 minute or until cheese melts.

7. Remove and place onto dinner plates.

8. Repeat process for remaining tortillas.

Preparation time: 20 minutes ● Servings: 2

Calories 365 ● Calories from Fat 67 ● Total Fat 7.5 g ● Saturated Fat 1.9 g ● Monounsaturated Fat 2.2 g ● Cholesterol 263 mg ● Sodium 418 mg ● Carbohydrate 29.4 g ● Dietary Fiber 4.0 g ● Sugars 0.7 g ● Protein 45.1 g

Exchanges: 2 starch, 5 lean meat

Black Bean and Tomato Salad

3/4 cup drained and rinsed canned black beans
1 cup fresh diced tomatoes
2 tablespoons reduced-fat oil and vinegar dressing ⚠
Salt and freshly ground black pepper

1. Place black beans and tomatoes in a bowl.
2. Add dressing and salt and pepper to taste. Toss well. Serve.

Preparation time: 5 minutes ● Servings: 2

Calories 112 ● Calories from Fat 13 ● Total Fat 1.5 g ● Saturated Fat 0.2 g ● Monounsaturated Fat 0.4 g ● Cholesterol 1 mg ● Sodium 9 mg ● Carbohydrate 19.5 g ● Dietary Fiber 6.7 g ● Sugars 3.1 g ● Protein 6.6 g

Exchanges: 1 starch, 1/2 fat

HELPFUL HINTS:

■ Diced fresh tomatoes can be found in the produce section of the supermarket.

■ Use two skillets to speed the cooking time of the quesadillas.

SHOPPING LIST

Seafood
10 ounces cooked, peeled medium shrimp

Dairy
1 small package shredded reduced-fat Cheddar cheese ⚠

Grocery
1 package 6-inch corn tortillas
1 can black beans

Produce
1/4 pound sliced, baby bello mushrooms
1 bag washed ready-to-eat spinach
1 container diced/chopped tomatoes

Staples
Olive oil spray
Reduced-fat oil and vinegar dressing ⚠
Salt
Black peppercorns

⚠ SHOP SMART!

Low-fat Cheddar cheese (per ounce): 49 calories, 2.0 g fat, 1.2 g saturated fat, 174 mg sodium

Reduced-fat vinaigrette or oil and vinegar dressing (per tablespoon): 11 calories, 1.0 g fat, 4 mg sodium

JERK SHRIMP WITH RICE AND PEAS

Scallions, thyme, allspice, and—most important of all—Scotch bonnet are the essential ingredients in jerk cooking. Jerking is a long process of spicing and cooking meat and fish over an open fire. We can enjoy jerk flavors without the long preparation and cooking times by using prepared jerk seasoning.

Rice and peas are an important part of Sunday lunch in Jamaica. This is a simple rice-and-peas dish to go with the Jerk Shrimp. Although it's not authentic, it captures the island flavor.

Jerk Shrimp

1 teaspoon canola oil
1/4 cup fresh diced onion
3/4 pound medium peeled shrimp
2 tablespoons light rum

1 tablespoon jerk seasoning
1 cup fresh diced tomatoes
Salt

COUNTDOWN

■ Start rice and peas.
■ Make shrimp.
■ Finish rice.

1. Heat oil in a medium nonstick skillet over medium-high heat.

2. Add onion, and sauté 2 minutes.

3. Add shrimp, rum, jerk seasoning, and tomatoes. Cook 2 minutes. Add salt to taste. Serve over Rice and Peas.

Preparation time: 5 minutes ● Servings: 2

Calories 262 ● Calories from Fat 49 ● Total Fat 5.5 g ● Saturated Fat 0.8 g ● Monounsaturated Fat 1.9 g ● Cholesterol 258 mg ● Sodium 266 mg ● Carbohydrate 10.3 g ● Dietary Fiber 2.4 g ● Sugars 3.7 g ● Protein 36 g

Exchanges: 1/2 carbohydrate, 5 lean meat

Rice and Peas

2 teaspoons canola oil
1/2 cup fresh diced onion
1/2 teaspoon minced garlic
1/2 cup long-grain white rice
1 cup fat-free low-sodium chicken broth
1/2 cup frozen petite peas
1 medium jalapeño pepper, seeded and chopped
Salt and freshly ground black pepper
2 scallions, sliced (1/3 cup)

1. Heat oil in a medium nonstick skillet, and sauté onion about 1 minute.

2. Add garlic and rice, and sauté 1 minute.

3. Add chicken broth. Bring to a simmer, cover, and let cook 10 minutes.

4. Add peas and jalapeño pepper. Cook another 5 minutes or until the rice is cooked through.

5. Add salt and pepper to taste. Sprinkle scallions on top. Serve.

Preparation time: 20 minutes ● Servings: 2

Calories 281 ● Calories from Fat 48 ● Total Fat 5.3 g ● Saturated Fat 0.5 g ● Monounsaturated Fat 3.0 g ● Cholesterol 0 mg ● Sodium 333 mg ● Carbohydrate 50.5 g ● Dietary Fiber 4.5 g ● Sugars 4.1 g ● Protein 8.1 g

Exchanges: 3 starch, 1 vegetable, 1/2 fat

SHOPPING LIST

Seafood
3/4 pound medium peeled shrimp

Grocery
1 bottle jerk seasoning
1 package long-grain white rice
1 package frozen petite peas
1 small bottle light rum

Produce
1 container diced fresh onion
1 container diced fresh tomatoes
1 medium jalapeño pepper
1 bunch scallions

Staples
Canola oil
Minced garlic
Fat-free low-sodium chicken broth
Salt
Black peppercorns

HELPFUL HINTS:

■ Diced fresh onions and tomato can be found in the produce section of the supermarket.

■ Minced garlic can be found in jars in the produce or condiment sections of the supermarket.

■ A quick way to slice scallions is to snip them with scissors.

■ Rum is called for in the Jerk Shrimp recipe. Water can be substituted.

■ Do not overcook the shrimp. They will become rubbery.

SPICY SHRIMP AND PEACH SALAD WITH LENTILS VINAIGRETTE

Plump juicy peaches, spicy shrimp, and vegetables create this colorful, refreshing salad supper. The contrast between hot and sweet flavors and soft and crunchy textures creates a mouthwatering dish that is easy to assemble and serve.

Spicy Shrimp and Peach Salad

1 ripe peach, cubed (1 cup)
1 medium red bell pepper, sliced (1 cup)
1/4 pound fresh snow peas, trimmed (about 1 cup)
3 tablespoons reduced-fat mayonnaise
1 tablespoon prepared horseradish

1 tablespoon Dijon mustard
10 ounces cooked shrimp, peeled and deveined
Salt and freshly ground black pepper
Several red leaf lettuce leaves

COUNTDOWN

■ Prepare all ingredients.
■ Make lentil salad.
■ Make sauce and finish shrimp salad.

1. Cut peach in half. Remove pit, and cut into 1-inch pieces.
2. Cut red pepper slices and snow peas into bite-size pieces, about the same size as the shrimp.
3. Mix mayonnaise, horseradish, and mustard together in a medium bowl. Add the shrimp, red pepper, and snow peas. Toss well. Add salt and pepper to taste.
4. Place lettuce leaves on two dinner plates and spoon salad on top. Sprinkle peach on top of salad.

Preparation time: 10 minutes ● Servings: 2

Calories 335 ● Calories from Fat 102 ● Total Fat 11.3 g ● Saturated Fat 1.8 g ● Monounsaturated Fat 2.5 g ● Cholesterol 266 mg ● Sodium 519 mg ● Carbohydrate 20.4 g ● Dietary Fiber 4.6 g ● Sugars 6.3 g ● Protein 37.8 g

Exchanges: 1 fruit, 1 vegetable, 5 lean meat, 1/2 fat

Lentils Vinaigrette

1 1/2 cups canned lentils, rinsed and drained ⚠️
1/2 cup chopped fresh cilantro
2 tablespoons reduced-fat vinaigrette dressing ⚠️
Salt and freshly ground black pepper

1. Place lentils, cilantro, and vinaigrette dressing in a bowl. Toss well. Add salt and pepper to taste. Serve.

Preparation time: 5 minutes ● Servings: 2

Calories 192 ● Calories from Fat 16 ● Total Fat 1.7 g ● Saturated Fat 0.2 g ● Monounsaturated Fat 0.5 g ● Cholesterol 1 mg ● Sodium 312 mg ● Carbohydrate 32.3 g ● Dietary Fiber 7.6 g ● Sugars 2.2 g ● Protein 12.2 g

Exchanges: 2 starch, 1 lean meat

HELPFUL HINTS:

■ Buy shelled, cooked shrimp from the fish or frozen food department of the supermarket.

■ Plums, nectarines, or mangoes can be used instead of peaches.

■ Basil, parsley, chives, or scallions can be used instead of cilantro for the lentil salad.

■ A quick way to chop cilantro is to wash, dry, and snip the leaves off the stem with scissors.

SHOPPING LIST

Seafood
10 ounces cooked shrimp, peeled and deveined

Grocery
1 bottle prepared horseradish
1 can lentils ⚠️

Produce
1 ripe peach
1 medium red bell pepper
1/4 pound fresh snow peas
1 small head red leaf lettuce
1 small bunch cilantro

Staples
Reduced-fat vinaigrette dressing ⚠️
Reduced-fat mayonnaise
Dijon mustard
Salt
Black peppercorns

⚠️ **SHOP SMART!**

Canned lentils (per cup): 240 calories, 680 mg sodium

Reduced-fat vinaigrette or oil and vinegar dressing (per tablespoon): 11 calories, 1.0 g fat, 4 mg sodium

HOT PEPPER SHRIMP WITH PIMENTO ENDIVE SALAD

Hot, spicy shrimp with lots of garlic is a popular tapas dish. By adding some thick country bread and a quick salad, it becomes an entire meal.

Belgian endive, sometimes called chicory, is a small cigar-shaped head of lettuce that is creamy white. It has tightly packed leaves and can be cleaned by wiping the outer leaves with a damp paper towel. The leaves will turn brown if soaked in water.

Hot Pepper Shrimp

2 large slices whole-grain country bread
2 teaspoons olive oil
Pinch crushed red pepper flakes
3/4 pound peeled shrimp

2 teaspoons minced garlic
2 tablespoons chopped fresh parsley (*optional*)
Salt and freshly ground black pepper

COUNTDOWN

■ Prepare ingredients.
■ Make salad.
■ Make shrimp.

1. Toast bread, and place on two dinner plates.
2. Heat a medium nonstick skillet over medium-high heat. Add olive oil and red pepper flakes.
3. When oil is hot, add shrimp and garlic. Toss shrimp in oil for 2–3 minutes or until shrimp are no longer translucent.
4. Remove from heat, and spoon over bread, including pan juices. Sprinkle with parsley (*optional*) and salt and pepper to taste.

Preparation time: 5 minutes ● Servings: 2

Calories 299 ● Calories from Fat 78 ● Total Fat 8.7 g ● Saturated Fat 1.4 g ● Monounsaturated Fat 3.9 g ● Cholesterol 258 mg ● Sodium 365 mg ● Carbohydrate 15.1 g ● Dietary Fiber 2.3 g ● Sugars 1.8 g ● Protein 38.5 g

Exchanges: 1 starch, 5 lean meat

Pimento Endive Salad

2 medium Belgian endive, sliced (about 2 cups)
1/2 cup canned pimento peppers, drained
1 cup Great Northern beans, rinsed and drained
1 tablespoon olive oil
Salt and freshly ground black pepper

1. Wipe endive with a damp paper towel. Cut off about 1/2 inch from the bottom or flat end and discard. Cut endive into 1/2-inch slices, and place in small salad bowl.

2. Cut pimentos into 1-inch strips and add to bowl, along with the beans.

3. Drizzle with olive oil, and add salt and pepper to taste. Toss well. Serve with the shrimp.

Preparation time: 5 minutes ● Servings: 2

Calories 229 ● Calories from Fat 68 ● Total Fat 7.6 g ● Saturated Fat 1.1 g ● Monounsaturated Fat 5.0 g ● Cholesterol 0 mg ● Sodium 16 mg ● Carbohydrate 31.5 g ● Dietary Fiber 8.3 g ● Sugars 1.9 g ● Protein 10.8 g

Exchanges: 1 1/2 starch, 1 vegetable, 1 lean meat, 1 fat

SHOPPING LIST

Seafood
3/4 pound peeled shrimp

Grocery
1 loaf whole-grain country bread
1 bottle crushed red pepper
1 jar/can pimentos
1 can Great Northern beans

Produce
1 small bunch parsley (*optional*)
2 medium Belgian endive

Staples
Olive oil
Minced garlic
Salt
Black peppercorns

HELPFUL HINTS:

■ Buy frozen peeled shrimp and keep it on hand for quick dinners.

■ Hot pepper sauce can be used instead of crushed red pepper.

■ Minced garlic can be found in jars in the produce or condiment sections of the supermarket.

■ Any type of lettuce can be used for the salad.

■ A quick way to chop parsley is to wash, dry, and snip the leaves right off the stem with scissors.

SHRIMP CAESAR SALAD

Classic Caesar Salad becomes a quick dinner when shrimp, pasta, and edamame beans are added. Crisp lettuce, crunchy beans, flavorful shrimp, and smooth, tangy dressing provide an enjoyable, mouthwatering combination.

Shrimp Caesar Salad

2 tablespoons broken walnuts (1/2 ounce)
2/3 cup whole-wheat penne pasta (2 ounces)
2 teaspoons olive oil
Salt and freshly ground black pepper
8 cups washed ready-to-eat Romaine lettuce

10 ounces cooked, peeled shrimp
1 cup frozen shelled edamame, thawed
  (or 1 cup shelled fresh)
4 tablespoons low-calorie Caesar dressing ⚡
2 tablespoons grated Parmesan cheese

COUNTDOWN

■ Preheat broiler.
■ Assemble dish.

1. Place a large saucepan filled with water on to boil over high heat.
2. Preheat broiler. Line a baking tray with foil. Place walnuts on tray, and toast under broiler 1 minute. Remove tray from broiler, remove walnuts, and set aside.
3. Cook pasta 8 minutes. Drain, leaving 2 tablespoons pasta water in pan. Add olive oil to saucepan. Return pasta to pan, along with salt and pepper to taste. Toss well.
4. Divide lettuce between two dinner plates.
5. Add pasta. Top with shrimp, walnuts, and edamame.
6. Drizzle dressing over salad.
7. Sprinkle Parmesan cheese on top.

Preparation time: 10 minutes ● Servings: 2

Calories 528 ● Calories from Fat 162 ● Total Fat 18.0 g ● Saturated Fat 2.9 g ● Monounsaturated Fat 5.2 g ● Cholesterol 262 mg ● Sodium 694 mg ● Carbohydrate 43.7 g ● Dietary Fiber 9.8 g ● Sugars 9.9 g ● Protein 51.2 g

Exchanges: 2 starch, 1 vegetable, 6 lean meat, 1 1/2 fat

HELPFUL HINTS:

- Any type of lettuce can be used.
- Toasting walnuts can be tricky. They burn quickly, so watch them.
- Pressed for time? Just add walnuts without toasting them.
- Defrost edamame for 30 seconds in a microwave oven or under warm tap water.

SHOPPING LIST

Seafood
10 ounces cooked, peeled shrimp

Dairy
1 small container grated Parmesan cheese

Grocery
1/2 ounce broken walnuts
1 package whole-wheat penne pasta
1 bag frozen shelled edamame
1 bottle low-calorie Caesar dressing **!**

Produce
1 bag washed ready-to-eat Romaine lettuce

Staples
Olive oil
Salt
Black peppercorns

! SHOP SMART!

Low-calorie Caesar salad dressing (per tablespoon): 16 calories, 0.7 g fat, 2.8 g carbohydrate, 172 mg sodium

PAN-SEARED SCALLOPS AND VEGETABLE MEDLEY RICE

Fresh sea scallops are served with a colorful Vegetable Medley Rice in this quick dinner that only takes 20 minutes to prepare. Scallops, which need very little cooking, should be prepared so that the inside remains creamy. Prolonged cooking will shrink and toughen them.

Sliced fresh onions, red bell pepper, and mushrooms are available in most produce sections of the supermarket. Using these cuts down on your prep time, and the rice can be made in 10 minutes.

Pan-Seared Scallops

3/4 pound fresh scallops
1 tablespoon olive oil

Salt and freshly ground black pepper
1 tablespoon dried chives

COUNTDOWN

■ Make rice dish.
■ Sauté scallops.

1. Rinse scallops in cool water. Drain, pat dry with a paper towel, and set aside.

2. Heat oil in the nonstick skillet used for the vegetables over high heat. When smoking, add scallops, and sauté for 1 minute; turn and sauté 2 minutes.

3. Add salt and pepper to taste. Sprinkle chives over scallops. Remove from skillet and serve.

Preparation time: 5 minutes ● Servings: 2

Calories 211 ● Calories from Fat 73 ● Total Fat 8.1 g ● Saturated Fat 1.1 g ● Monounsaturated Fat 5.0 g ● Cholesterol 54 mg ● Sodium 276 mg ● Carbohydrate 4.2 g ● Dietary Fiber 0.1 g ● Sugars 0.1 g ● Protein 28.7 g

Exchanges: 4 lean meat, 1/2 fat

Vegetable Medley Rice

1 package microwaveable brown rice (for 1 cup cooked)
1/2 cup nonfat plain yogurt
1 tablespoon prepared horseradish
1 tablespoon olive oil
1 cup fresh sliced onion
1 cup fresh diced red bell pepper
1 cup sliced mushrooms
Salt and freshly ground black pepper

1. Cook rice according to package instructions, and measure 1 cup cooked rice. Reserve the rest for a later use.

2. Meanwhile, mix yogurt and horseradish together in a medium bowl.

3. Add cooked rice to bowl. Set aside.

4. Heat oil in a nonstick skillet over medium-high heat. Add onion, red bell pepper, and mushrooms. Sauté 5 minutes. Add to the bowl with the rice. Add salt and pepper to taste. Toss well. Serve.

Preparation time: 10 minutes ● Servings: 2

Calories 280 ● Calories from Fat 81 ● Total Fat 9.0 g ● Saturated Fat 1.3 g ● Monounsaturated Fat 5.5 g ● Cholesterol 1 mg ● Sodium 86 mg ● Carbohydrate 38.2 g ● Dietary Fiber 4.5 g ● Sugars 7.1 g ● Protein 8.8 g

Exchanges: 2 starch, 2 vegetable, 1 1/2 fat

HELPFUL HINTS:

■ Scallops should smell sweet, not be sitting in liquid, and show no browning when purchased.

■ Sliced fresh onion can be found in the produce section of the supermarket.

■ Diced fresh bell peppers can be found in the produce section of the supermarket.

■ Sauté the vegetables in a skillet and remove. Use the same skillet to cook the scallops.

SHOPPING LIST

Seafood
3/4 pound fresh scallops

Dairy
1 carton nonfat plain yogurt

Grocery
1 bottle dried chives
1 package microwaveable brown rice
1 bottle prepared horseradish

Produce
1 container fresh sliced onion
1 container fresh diced red bell pepper
1 package slice mushrooms

Staples
Olive oil
Salt
Black peppercorns

CURRY-KISSED SCALLOPS WITH CARROTS AND RICE

Sweet scallops touched by a dusting of curry are the centerpiece of this light and quick meal. There's no chopping or slicing.

The curry powder sold in supermarkets is a blend of about 15 herbs, spices, and seeds. This type of powder loses its flavor quickly. If you have curry powder that is more than six months old, buy a new one. It will add more flavors to the dish.

Curry-Kissed Scallops

3/4 pound sea scallops
2 teaspoons curry powder
1 tablespoon olive oil
Salt and freshly ground black pepper

1/4 cup water
2 tablespoons apricot jam
6 tablespoons fat-free half and half
2 tablespoons scallions

COUNTDOWN

■ Make rice and cover while scallops cook.
■ Make scallops.

1. Rinse, drain, and pat scallops dry with a paper towel.

2. Toss the scallops in the curry powder, making sure all sides are coated.

3. Heat oil in a nonstick skillet over high heat.

4. Add scallops to pan and sauté 1 minute; turn and sauté 2 minutes. Add salt and pepper to taste.

5. Transfer scallops to a bowl. Add water and apricot jam to the skillet; simmer 30 seconds, stirring to melt jam.

6. Add half and half, and simmer 1 minute or until sauce thickens.

7. Spoon sauce over scallops. Sprinkle scallions on top and serve.

Preparation time: 10 minutes ● Servings: 2

Calories 292 ● Calories from Fat 81 ● Total Fat 9.0 g ● Saturated Fat 1.5 g ● Monounsaturated Fat 5.3 g ● Cholesterol 56 mg ● Sodium 348 mg ● Carbohydrate 22.3 g ● Dietary Fiber 1.0 g ● Sugars 11.0 g ● Protein 30.2 g

Exchanges: 1 1/2 carbohydrate, 4 lean meat, 1/2 fat

Carrots and Rice

1 cup water
1 cup 10-minute brown rice (to yield 1 1/2 cups cooked rice)
1/2 cup shredded carrots
1 tablespoon olive oil
Salt and freshly ground black pepper

1. Bring water to a boil in a saucepan. Add rice and carrots. Return to a boil, lower heat to medium, cover, and cook 5 minutes.

2. Remove from heat, stir, cover, and let rest 5 minutes.

3. Add oil and salt and pepper to taste and serve.

Preparation time: 15 minutes ● Servings: 2

Calories 221 ● Calories from Fat 75 ● Total Fat 8.3 g ● Saturated Fat 1.2 g ● Monounsaturated Fat 5.4 g ● Cholesterol 0 mg ● Sodium 29 mg ● Carbohydrate 36.6 g ● Dietary Fiber 2.8 g ● Sugars 1.3 g ● Protein 3.3 g

Exchanges: 2 starches, 1 vegetable, 1 fat

SHOPPING LIST

Seafood
3/4 pound sea scallops

Dairy
1 small carton fat-free half and half

Grocery
1 jar curry powder
1 small bottle apricot jam
1 10-minute box brown rice

Produce
1 small bunch scallions
1 bag shredded carrots

Staples
Olive oil
Salt
Black peppercorns

HELPFUL HINTS:

■ Shredded or matchstick carrots can be found in the produce section of the market.

■ Make sure skillet is hot enough to sear scallops.

■ If using smaller bay scallops, sauté 2 minutes, tossing the scallops to cook all sides.

■ A simple way to turn scallops in the skillet is with tongs.

PESTO SCALLOPS WITH FRESH FETTUCCINI

Pesto sauce, made with basil and parsley, lends a fresh, herbal flavor to scallops. I keep a bag of frozen sea scallops on hand for quick dinners. They take only a few minutes to defrost in a bowl of cold water. This dish takes only 5 minutes to make if you're using prepared pesto sauce.

Pesto Scallops

Olive oil spray
3/4 pound sea scallops

2 tablespoons reduced-fat pesto sauce ⚡
2 tablespoons pine nuts

COUNTDOWN
- Place a large pot of water for fettuccini on to boil.
- Prepare ingredients.
- Make fettuccini.
- Make scallops.

1. Heat a nonstick skillet over medium-high heat, and spray with olive oil spray.
2. Add scallops and sauté 3 minutes; turn and sauté 2 minutes.
3. Remove from heat, and add pesto sauce. Toss well.
4. Divide between two dinner plates, and sprinkle pine nuts over scallops. Serve with fettucini.

Preparation time: 7 minutes ● Servings: 2

Calories 293 ● Calories from Fat 107 ● Total Fat 11.9 g ● Saturated Fat 2.0 g ● Monounsaturated Fat 5.7 g ● Cholesterol 58 mg ● Sodium 413 mg ● Carbohydrate 7.9 g ● Dietary Fiber 0.9 g ● Sugars 1.3g ● Protein 32.4 g

Exchanges: 1/2 carbohydrate, 5 lean meat, 1 fat

Fresh Fettuccini

1/4 pound fresh whole-wheat fettuccini (1 1/2 cups cooked)
1 tablespoon olive oil
1 cup fresh diced tomatoes
Salt and freshly ground black pepper

1. Bring a large saucepan filled with water to a boil over high heat. Add fettuccini, and cook 3 minutes or according to package instructions.
2. Transfer 2 tablespoons cooking liquid to a medium bowl. Add the olive oil, and mix well.
3. Drain the fettuccini, and add to the bowl. Add the tomato cubes and salt and pepper to taste. Toss well and serve.

Preparation time: 10 minutes ● Servings: 2

Calories 274 ● Calories from Fat 70 ● Total Fat 7.7 g ● Saturated Fat 1.1 g ● Monounsaturated Fat 5.1 g ● Cholesterol 0 mg ● Sodium 10 mg ● Carbohydrate 46.3 g ● Dietary Fiber 5.8 g ● Sugars 4.5 g ● Protein 9.1 g

Exchanges: 2 1/2 starch, 1 vegetable, 1 fat

HELPFUL HINTS:

■ Diced fresh tomatoes can be found in the produce section of the supermarket.

■ Prepared pesto sauce can be found in the deli section or in jars in the condiment section of the market.

■ Diced fresh tomatoes can be found in the produce section of the supermarket.

■ Whole-wheat spaghetti or linguine can be used instead of fettuccini.

SHOPPING LIST

Seafood
3/4 pound sea scallops

Grocery
1 container reduced-fat pesto sauce **!**
1 package pine nuts
4 ounces whole-wheat fresh fettuccini

Produce
1 container fresh diced tomatoes

Staples
Olive oil spray
Olive oil
Salt
Black peppercorns

! SHOP SMART!

Reduced-fat pesto sauce (per tablespoon): 80 calories, 4.8 g total fat, 1 g saturated fat, 135 mg sodium [*Example*: Buitoni Reduced-Fat Pesto with Basil]

CRAB SCAMPI AND SPAGHETTI

To Italians, scampi is a small lobster called a prawn. However, in America, scampi is a term for the sauce that goes with seafood. Jumbo lump crab in a garlic-wine sauce is a new take on this traditional Italian dish. Serve the crab sauce over spaghetti, and enjoy a quick Italian seafood dinner.

Crab Scampi

2 teaspoons olive oil

2 teaspoons minced garlic

3/4 cup dry vermouth

2 teaspoons Worcestershire sauce

1 cup drained low-sodium canned diced tomatoes ⚠

Several drops hot pepper sauce

3/4 pound canned or frozen jumbo lump crabmeat (about 2 1/2 cups)

1/2 cup fresh parsley, chopped (*optional*)

Salt and freshly ground black pepper

COUNTDOWN

■ Place water for spaghetti on to boil.

■ Make scampi.

■ Cook spaghetti.

1. Heat olive oil in a nonstick skillet over medium-high heat. Add garlic, vermouth, Worcestershire sauce, tomatoes, and hot pepper sauce. Cook 2 minutes to blend flavors.

2. Add crabmeat. Toss for 2 minutes to warm crabmeat, stirring occasionally.

3. Sprinkle with parsley (*optional*) and salt and pepper to taste. Serve over spaghetti.

Preparation time: 10 minutes ● Servings: 2

Calories 292 ● Calories from Fat 60 ● Total Fat 6.7 g ● Saturated Fat 1.1 g ● Monounsaturated Fat 3.7 g ● Cholesterol 132 mg ● Sodium 588 mg ● Carbohydrate 9.3 g ● Dietary Fiber 1.9 g ● Sugars 3.6 g ● Protein 32.5 g

Exchanges: 1 vegetable, 5 lean meat, 1/2 alcohol

Spaghetti

1/4 pound whole-wheat thin spaghetti
2 teaspoons olive oil
Salt and freshly ground black pepper

1. Bring a large saucepan with 3–4 quarts water to a boil over high heat. Add spaghetti, and boil 8–9 minutes.

2. Remove 2 tablespoons cooking water and reserve.

3. Drain spaghetti, and place back in saucepan with reserved water and olive oil. Toss well. Add pepper to taste. Toss and divide between two dinner plates.

Preparation time: 10 minutes ● Servings: 2

Calories 238 ● Calories from Fat 48 ● Total Fat 5.3 g ● Saturated Fat 0.8 g ● Monounsaturated Fat 3.4 g ● Cholesterol 0 mg ● Sodium 5 mg ● Carbohydrate 42.8 g ● Dietary Fiber 4.7 g ● Sugars 2.1 g ● Protein 8.3 g

Exchanges: 3 starch

HELPFUL HINTS:

■ Look for canned or frozen jumbo lump crab. Backfin crab can be substituted.

■ This recipe will also work with imitation crabmeat.

■ Minced garlic can be found in jars in the produce or condiment sections of the supermarket.

■ The quickest way to chop parsley and basil is to snip the leaves with scissors.

SHOPPING LIST

Seafood
3/4 ounces canned or frozen jumbo lump crabmeat

Grocery
1 small bottle dry vermouth
1 small bottle Worcestershire sauce
1/4 pound whole-wheat spaghetti
1 can low-sodium diced tomatoes **!**
1 bottle hot pepper sauce

Produce
1 small bunch parsley (*optional*)

Staples
Olive oil
Minced garlic
Salt
Black peppercorns

! SHOP SMART!

Canned low-sodium diced tomatoes (per cup): 41 calories, 9.6 g carbohydrate, 24 mg sodium

SPAGHETTI WITH CLAMS AND HERB SAUCE AND ITALIAN SALAD

Spaghetti with clam sauce is fresh, flavorful, and easy to make. When buying clams, look for shells that are tightly closed. At home, tap any shells that are open. The clams should close; if not, discard them. Store clams in the refrigerator loosely covered with a clean towel. Use them within one or two days. Scrub the shells under cold water before cooking them. Complete the meal with a fresh Italian salad.

Spaghetti with Clams and Herb Sauce

1/4 pound whole-wheat spaghetti (1 1/2 cups cooked)
2 tablespoons olive oil, divided
2 teaspoons minced garlic
1/3 cup bottled clam juice
2 pounds clams (steamers or medium clams)

2 cups fresh diced tomatoes
1/3 cup sliced scallions
1/4 cup snipped fresh basil leaves
Salt and freshly ground black pepper

COUNTDOWN

■ Place water for pasta on to boil.
■ Prepare clams.
■ Cook pasta.
■ Cook clams.
■ Make the salad.

1. Bring a large pot of water to a boil. Add the spaghetti, and cook according to the package directions until al dente. Drain, toss with 1 tablespoon olive oil, and set aside.

2. Heat remaining 1 tablespoon olive oil in a nonstick skillet over low heat. Add the garlic, and cook, stirring occasionally, 1 minute.

3. Add the clam juice. Cover with a lid, raise the heat to medium-low, and simmer for 1 minute to blend the flavors.

4. Add the clams. Cover and simmer, shaking the pan, until they open, about 5 minutes. Discard any clams that do not open.

5. Transfer clams and their juices to a large bowl. Add the tomatoes and scallions to the bowl and toss. Sprinkle with basil. Add salt and pepper to taste. Toss lightly to combine.

6. Divide the spaghetti between two shallow bowls. Top with the clam sauce. Serve immediately.

Preparation time: 15 minutes ● Servings: 2

Calories 449 ● Calories from Fat 144 ● Total Fat 16.0 g ● Saturated Fat 2.2 g ● Monounsaturated Fat 10.1g ● Cholesterol 38 mg ● Sodium 267 mg ● Carbohydrate 56.1 g ● Dietary Fiber 7.6 g ● Sugars 7.3 g ● Protein 25.3 g

Exchanges: 3 starch, 1 vegetable, 2 lean meat, 2 fat

Italian Salad

4 cups washed ready-to-eat Italian-style salad
2 tablespoons reduced-fat Italian dressing ▮

1. Place salad in a bowl, and toss with the dressing. Serve.

Preparation time: 2 minutes ● Servings: 2

Calories 27 ● Calories from Fat 11 ● Total Fat 1.2 g ● Saturated Fat 0.1 g
● Monounsaturated Fat 0.3g ● Cholesterol 1 mg ● Sodium 12 mg
● Carbohydrate 3.8 g ● Dietary Fiber 2.0 g ● Sugars 1.8 g ● Protein 1.2 g

Exchanges: 1 vegetable

HELPFUL HINTS:

■ Mussels can be used instead of clams.

■ Diced fresh tomatoes can be found in the produce section of the supermarket.

■ Minced garlic can be found in jars in the produce section of the market.

■ A quick way to chop fresh herbs and to slice scallions is to snip them with scissors.

SHOPPING LIST

Seafood
2 pounds clams (steamers or medium clams)

Grocery
1 bottle clam juice
1/4 pound whole-wheat spaghetti

Produce
1 container fresh diced tomatoes
1 bunch scallions
1 small bunch fresh basil
1 bag washed ready-to-eat salad

Staples
Olive oil
Minced garlic
Reduced-fat Italian (oil and vinegar, not creamy) dressing ▮
Salt
Black peppercorns

▮ SHOP SMART!

Reduced-fat Italian dressing—oil and vinegar, not creamy dressing (per tablespoon): 11 calories, 1.0 g fat, 4 mg sodium

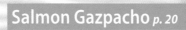

Sweet and Sour Shrimp
with Brown Rice *p. 56*

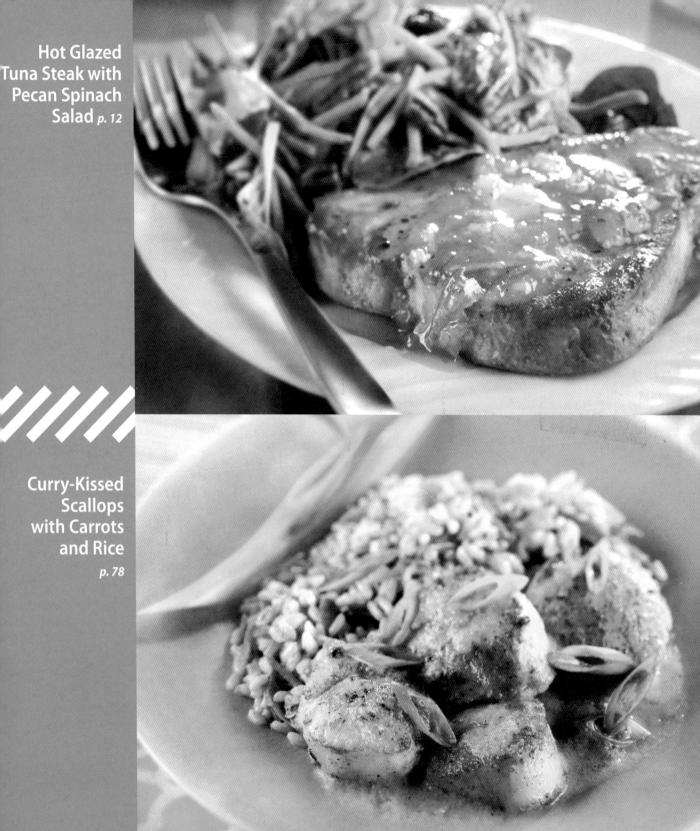

Hot Glazed Tuna Steak with Pecan Spinach Salad *p. 12*

Curry-Kissed Scallops with Carrots and Rice

p. 78

Grilled Chicken Wraps and
Parmesan Corn *p. 120*

Chili Chicken with
Southwestern Barley Salad *p. 96*

Balsamic Pork Scaloppini with
Garlic Sweet Potatoes and
Sugar Snap Peas *p. 158*

Brandied Apples and
Pork with Egg Noodles *p. 162*

Vietnamese Hot and Spicy
Stir-Fry Beef and Chinese Noodles
with Snow Peas *p. 232*

POULTRY

Aga Khan's Chicken Curry and Rice 88

Almond-Grape Chicken Salad with Crunchy Coleslaw 90

Basque Chicken with Saffron Rice 92

Black Bean Chicken Chili and Iceberg Salad 94

Chili Chicken with Southwestern Barley Salad 96

Chicken Pizzaioli with Fennel and Bean Salad 98

Chicken Tostadas and Cilantro Tomatoes 100

Chicken and Garlic Greens with Spicy Sautéed Potatoes 102

Chicken and Shiitake Yakitori 104

Chicken and Walnuts in Lettuce Puffs with Chinese Rice 106

Chinese Salad with Asian Dressing 108

Coq au Vin (Chicken Stewed in Red Wine) with Brown Rice 110

Country Mushroom and Sausage Soup with Onion-Garlic Crostini 112

Crispy Chicken with Ratatouille (Sautéed Provençal Vegetables) 114

Curried Chicken Pot Pie 116

Dijon Chicken with Vegetable Quinoa 118

Grilled Chicken Wraps and Parmesan Corn 120

Hawaiian Chicken with Pineapple Salad 122

Honey-Spiced Mock Chicken Wings and Celery with Blue Cheese Dressing 124

Indian-Spiced Chicken with Cumin-Scented Rice and Spinach 126

Chicken Diavolo (Italian Chicken in Spicy Tomato Sauce) with Zucchini Carrot Gratinée 128

Jacques Pepin's Supreme of Chicken with Balsamic Vinegar and Onion Sauce with Corn and Peas 130

Marsala-Glazed Chicken with Roman Spinach 132

Mexican Sope (Layered Open Tortilla Sandwich) 134

Pistachio-Crusted Chicken and Broccoli Farfalle 136

Poached Chicken with Fresh Tomato Mayonnaise Sauce and Cucumber Rice Salad 138

Pollo Tonnato (Chicken in Tuna Sauce) 140

Sherry Chicken and Green Bean Pimento Rice 142

Tarragon Chicken with Orzo and Chives 144

Thai Chicken Kabobs with Brown Rice 146

Turkey and Apple Salad with Herbed Cheese Crostini 148

Turkey Normandy with Sweet Potatoes 150

Turkey Picadillo with Brown Rice 152

Turkey Stroganoff with Egg Noodles 154

AGA KHAN'S CHICKEN CURRY AND RICE

While at Le Cordon Bleu culinary school, I learned about this aromatic and gently spicy chicken curry that the school had developed for the Aga Khan. It became his favorite curry dinner. That dish inspired this recipe.

The curry powder that we buy is actually a combination of many spices. The spices for an authentic curry are blended just before use. I use mild curry powder here to preserve the delicate blend of flavors. If you like your curry hot, use the hot curry powder.

Aga Khan's Chicken Curry

1 1/2 pounds chicken breasts on the bone, without wings, skin removed (to yield 3/4 pound meat)

2 teaspoons canola oil

1/2 cup fresh diced onion

1 teaspoon minced garlic

1 teaspoon ground cinnamon

1/8 teaspoon cayenne pepper

1/2 tablespoon mild curry powder

1 Golden Delicious apple, cored and sliced (about 2 cups)

2 cups green beans, trimmed, cut into 1-inch pieces

3 ounces (approximately 1/3 cup) canned light coconut milk ⬛

1/2 cup water

1 cup fresh diced tomatoes

1 teaspoon cornstarch

1 1/2 tablespoons half and half

1 tablespoon bottled lemon juice

Salt and freshly ground black pepper

COUNTDOWN

- Place water for rice on to boil.
- Prepare ingredients.
- Make rice.
- Make chicken.
- Complete the recipe.

1. Cut chicken breasts into 4 pieces each (unless you've already had the butcher do this).

2. Heat oil in a nonstick skillet over medium-high heat. Add chicken, flesh side down, and brown for 2 minutes.

3. Turn chicken over, add the onion and garlic, and sauté without browning, 3 minutes.

4. Stir in the cinnamon, cayenne pepper, and curry powder for about 30 seconds to release their oils.

5. Add the apple slices, and cook 30 seconds.

6. Add beans, coconut milk, and water, and bring to a simmer. Lower heat to medium, cover with foil, and then with a lid. Simmer 15 minutes. Add the tomatoes.

7. Mix cornstarch with half and half, and add to skillet. Simmer 5 minutes. Add lemon juice and salt and pepper to taste. Serve over rice.

Preparation time: 30 minutes ● Servings: 2

Calories 418 ● Calories from Fat 121 ● Total Fat 13.5 g ● Saturated Fat 3.7 g ● Monounsaturated Fat 4.65 g ● Cholesterol 113 mg ● Sodium 230 mg ● Carbohydrate 38.4 g ● Dietary Fiber 9.7 g ● Sugars 18.4 g ● Protein 40.9 g

Exchanges: 1 fruit, 2 vegetable, 1/2 carbohydrate, 5 lean meat, 1 fat

Rice

1/4 cup white long-grain rice
Salt and freshly ground black pepper

1. Bring a large saucepan filled with water to a boil over high heat. Add rice, and boil 10 minutes.

2. Drain and add salt and pepper to taste.

3. Place rice on two dinner plates, and serve chicken and sauce over top.

Preparation time: 15 minutes ● Servings: 2

Calories 84 ● Calories from Fat 1 ● Total Fat 0.2 g ● Saturated Fat 0 g ● Monounsaturated Fat 0.1 g ● Cholesterol 0 mg ● Sodium 1 mg ● Carbohydrate 18.5 g ● Dietary Fiber 0.3 g ● Sugars 0 g ● Protein 1.7 g

Exchanges: 1 starch

HELPFUL HINTS:

■ This meal tastes even better the second day. If time permits, double the recipe and save half for another meal.

■ Ask butcher to cut each chicken breast into quarters.

■ Diced fresh onions and tomatoes can be found in the produce section of the supermarket.

■ Buy trimmed beans.

■ Foil is placed over the chicken and then the pot is covered with a lid. This keeps the moisture in the dish.

SHOPPING LIST

Poultry
1 1/2 pounds chicken breasts on the bone, without wings

Dairy
1 small carton half and half

Grocery
1 bottle ground cinnamon
1 bottle cayenne pepper
1 bottle mild curry powder
1 can light coconut milk ⚡
1 bottle lemon juice
1 package white long-grain rice

Produce
1 container fresh diced onion
1 container fresh diced tomatoes
1 golden delicious apple
1 package trimmed green beans

Staples
Canola oil
Minced garlic
Cornstarch
Salt
Black peppercorns

⚡ **SHOP SMART!**

Light coconut milk (per 1/4 cup): 34 calories, 3.3 g fat, 1.9 g saturated fat, 2.3 g carbohydrate, 15 mg sodium

ALMOND-GRAPE CHICKEN SALAD WITH CRUNCHY COLESLAW

The only heat you need for this quick summer meal is a microwave oven. It's a simple way to "poach" chicken. The chicken is placed on a plate, covered with another plate, and microwaved for 4 minutes. This method produces cooked chicken that is tender and juicy.

Almond-Grape Chicken Salad

2 tablespoons reduced-fat mayonnaise
2 tablespoons nonfat plain yogurt
3/4 pound boneless, skinless chicken breasts
1 cup seedless grapes
Salt and freshly ground black pepper

Several washed ready-to-eat lettuce leaves
2 tablespoons sliced almonds
2 tablespoons fresh snipped chives or
   2 teaspoons dried chives

COUNTDOWN

■ Make coleslaw and set aside to marinate while making chicken salad.
■ Make chicken salad.

1. Mix mayonnaise and yogurt in a bowl. Set aside.
2. Place chicken on a microwave-safe plate, and cover with a second plate. Microwave on high 4 minutes. Remove and let stand, covered, for 2 minutes. A meat thermometer should read 165°F.
3. Cut chicken into 1/2-inch pieces. Add chicken and grapes to the bowl. Mix well. Add salt and pepper to taste.
4. Divide lettuce leaves between two plates, and spoon chicken on top.
5. Sprinkle almonds and chives over chicken, and serve.

Preparation time: 10 minutes ● Servings: 2

Calories 358 ● Calories from Fat 127 ● Total Fat 14.1 g ● Saturated Fat 2.2 g ● Monounsaturated Fat 5.5 g ● Cholesterol 113 mg ● Sodium 314 mg ● Carbohydrate 18.6 g ● Dietary Fiber 2.2 g ● Sugars 13.1 g ● Protein 39.9 g

Exchanges: 1 fruit, 6 lean meat, 1 fat

Crunchy Coleslaw

2 tablespoons reduced-fat mayonnaise
1 tablespoon white distilled vinegar
Sugar substitute to equal 1/2 teaspoon sugar
2 cups shredded ready-to-eat coleslaw mix
Salt and freshly ground black pepper
2 slices whole-grain bread (1 ounce each)

1. Mix mayonnaise, vinegar, and sugar substitute together in a bowl.

2. Add coleslaw mixture, and toss well. Add salt and pepper to taste.

3. Serve with bread on the side or make an open-face sandwich with the chicken salad and coleslaw.

Preparation time: 5 minutes ● Servings: 2

Calories 139 ● Calories from Fat 54 ● Total Fat 6.0 g ● Saturated Fat 1.0 g ● Monounsaturated Fat 1.7 g ● Cholesterol 5 mg ● Sodium 246 mg ● Carbohydrate 17.1 g ● Dietary Fiber 3.7 g ● Sugars 4.5 g ● Protein 4.7 g

Exchanges: 1 starch, 1 fat

HELPFUL HINTS:

■ A simple way to chop chives is to cut them with scissors.

SHOPPING LIST

Poultry
3/4 pound boneless, skinless chicken breasts

Dairy
1 small carton nonfat plain yogurt

Grocery
1 small package sliced almonds
1 bottle white distilled vinegar
1 loaf whole-grain bread

Produce
1 small container seedless grapes
1 bag washed ready-to-eat lettuce leaves
1 bunch chives
1 bag shredded ready-to-eat coleslaw mix

Staples
Sugar substitute
Reduced-fat mayonnaise
Salt
Black peppercorns

BASQUE CHICKEN WITH SAFFRON RICE

The combination of onion, tomato, garlic, and red pepper is used in many cuisines. The Spanish call it *sofrito*. In the Basque region of Spain, sofrito includes lots of red pepper and some hot peppers.

Pilaf (sometimes called pilau) is a rice dish that begins with first sautéing rice and then cooking it in broth. This can be done in the oven or on a burner.

Saffron Rice

1 teaspoon olive oil
1/4 cup fresh sliced onion
1/2 cup long-grain white rice

1 1/2 cups water
1/8 teaspoon saffron threads
Salt and freshly ground black pepper

COUNTDOWN

- Start rice.
- Prepare remaining ingredients.
- Prepare chicken.
- Finish rice.

1. Heat oil in a nonstick skillet over medium-high heat. Add onion and rice. Sauté 2 minutes, stirring several times.
2. Add water and saffron. Bring to a boil, reduce heat to medium, cover with a lid, and cook 10 minutes. Remove lid, stir the rice, and add salt and pepper to taste. Serve.

Preparation time: 15 minutes ● Servings: 2

Calories 195 ● Calories from Fat 23 ● Total Fat 2.6 g ● Saturated Fat 0.4 g ● Monounsaturated Fat 1.7 g ● Cholesterol 0 mg ● Sodium 3 mg ● Carbohydrate 38.4 g ● Dietary Fiber 0.9 g ● Sugars 0.7 g ● Protein 3.5 g

Exchanges: 2 1/2 starch

Basque Chicken

2 teaspoons olive oil
3/4 pound boneless, skinless chicken breasts
1/2 cup fresh sliced onion
1/2 cup lean deli ham, cut into 1/4-inch strips (2 ounces) ▮
1 cup canned low-sodium diced tomatoes, drained ▮
3/4 cup drained, canned sliced pimentos
Several drops hot pepper sauce
Salt and freshly ground black pepper

1. Heat olive oil in a nonstick skillet over medium-high heat. Add chicken, and brown 2 minutes; turn and brown 2 more minutes. Transfer to a plate.

2. Add onion, ham, and tomatoes to skillet. Sauté 5 minutes.

3. Return chicken to skillet. Add pimentos and hot pepper sauce. Lower heat to medium, cover with a lid, and cook 4 minutes. A meat thermometer should read 165°F.

4. Add salt and pepper to taste. Serve chicken over rice, and spoon sauce on top.

Preparation time: 12 minutes ● Servings: 2

Calories 311 ● Calories from Fat 90 ● Total Fat 10.0 g ● Saturated Fat 1.8 g ● Monounsaturated Fat 4.9 g ● Cholesterol 121 mg ● Sodium 530 mg ● Carbohydrate 11.4 g ● Dietary Fiber 3.1 g ● Sugars 6.0 g ● Protein 43.5 g

Exchanges: 2 vegetable, 6 lean meat

HELPFUL HINTS:

■ Rotisserie or roasted chicken can be used. Remove skin and fat before adding to the sauce.

■ If sliced pimentos aren't available, cut whole ones into 1/4-inch strips.

■ Turmeric or bijol can be used instead of saffron.

■ Sliced fresh onions can be found in the produce section of the supermarket.

SHOPPING LIST

Poultry
3/4 pound boneless, skinless chicken breasts

Deli
1 small package lean ham (2 ounces needed) ▮

Grocery
1 package long-grain white rice
1 small package saffron threads
1 can low-sodium diced tomatoes ▮
1 can/jar sliced pimentos

Produce
1 container fresh sliced onion

Staples
Olive oil
Hot pepper sauce
Salt
Black peppercorns

▮ SHOP SMART!

Lean ham (per ounce): 30 calories, 0.7 g fat, 0.2 g saturated fat, 301 mg sodium

Canned low-sodium diced tomatoes (per cup): 41 calories, 9.6 g carbohydrate, 24 mg sodium

BLACK BEAN CHICKEN CHILI AND ICEBERG SALAD

This quick 15-minute black bean chicken chili combines Latin and Southwestern flavors. The directions are for two servings, but this chili is perfect for a casual dinner with friends. You can increase the ingredient amounts as desired.

Black Bean Chicken Chili

1 teaspoon olive oil

3/4 pound boneless, skinless chicken breast, cut into 1/2-inch cubes

1 1/2 cups fresh diced onion, divided

1 teaspoon minced garlic

1 cup canned black beans, rinsed and drained

1 cup frozen corn kernels

1 1/2 tablespoons chili powder

1 teaspoon ground cumin

2 cups canned low-sodium diced tomatoes ⬛

Salt and freshly ground black pepper

1/4 cup shredded reduced-fat Mexican-style cheese (1 ounce) ⬛

1/4 cup chopped cilantro (*garnish*)

COUNTDOWN

■ Start chili.

■ While chili cooks, assemble salad.

1. Heat oil in a large nonstick skillet over medium-high heat. Add chicken. Brown for 1 minute, tossing as cubes brown.

2. Add 1 cup onion, and sauté 1 minute.

3. Add garlic, black beans, corn, chili powder, cumin, and diced tomatoes. Bring to a simmer and then lower heat to medium. Cover with a lid, and simmer 10 minutes.

4. Add salt and pepper to taste. Add more chili powder or cumin as needed.

5. Spoon into two large bowls, and sprinkle cheese on top.

6. Place remaining 1/2 cup onion and cilantro in separate bowls and serve with the chili.

Preparation time: 20 minutes ● Servings: 2

Calories 526 ● Calories from Fat 104 ● Total Fat 11.3 g ● Saturated Fat 3.4 g ● Monounsaturated Fat 4.2 g ● Cholesterol 117 mg ● Sodium 355 mg ● Carbohydrate 56.8 g ● Dietary Fiber 13.7 g ● Sugars 15.5 g ● Protein 53.2 g

Exchanges: 2 1/2 starch, 3 vegetable, 6 lean meat

Iceberg Salad

2 large wedges of iceberg lettuce (about 4 cups)
2 tablespoons reduced-fat vinaigrette dressing ⚠

1. Place iceberg on two small salad plates. Drizzle 1 tablespoon dressing over each wedge and serve.

Preparation time: 2 minutes ● Servings: 2

Calories 27 ● Calories from Fat 11 ● Total Fat 1.2 g ● Saturated Fat 0.1 g ● Monounsaturated Fat 0.3 g ● Cholesterol 1 mg ● Sodium 12 mg ● Carbohydrate 3.8 g ● Dietary Fiber 2.0 g ● Sugars 1.8 g ● Protein 1.2 g

Exchanges: 1 vegetable

HELPFUL HINTS:

■ Any type of lettuce can be used for the salad.

■ Diced fresh onions can be found in the produce section of the supermarket.

SHOPPING LIST

Deli
3/4 pound boneless, skinless chicken breast

Dairy
1 small package shredded reduced-fat Mexican-style cheese ⚠

Grocery
1 large can low-sodium diced tomatoes ⚠
1 bottle chili powder
1 bottle ground cumin
1 can black beans
1 package frozen corn kernels

Produce
1 container fresh diced onion
1 head iceberg lettuce
1 bunch cilantro

Staples
Olive oil
Reduced-fat vinaigrette dressing ⚠
Minced garlic
Salt
Black peppercorns

⚠ SHOP SMART!

Canned low-sodium diced tomatoes (per cup): 41 calories, 9.6 g carbohydrate, 24 mg sodium

Reduced-fat vinaigrette or oil and vinegar dressing (per tablespoon): 11 calories, 1.0 g fat, 4 mg sodium

Reduced-fat Mexican-style cheese (per ounce; 1/4 cup): 80 calories, 5.5 g fat, 3.3 g saturated fat, 220 mg sodium

CHILI CHICKEN WITH SOUTHWESTERN BARLEY SALAD

This Chili Chicken is full of hot, spicy Southwestern flavors and is served over a bed of lettuce with Green Onion Dressing. The side dish is made with barley, a versatile cereal grain with a rich, nutlike flavor and an appealing chewy, pasta-like consistency.

Chili Chicken

1/2 cup fresh diced onion
1 teaspoon minced garlic
1 tablespoon chili powder
1 teaspoon ground cumin
1/8 teaspoon salt
1/8 teaspoon freshly ground black pepper

2 6-ounce boneless, skinless chicken breasts
3 cups washed ready-to-eat Romaine lettuce
1 medium tomato, cut into 8 wedges
2 tablespoons reduced-fat oil and vinegar dressing
2 tablespoons sliced scallions

COUNTDOWN
- Preheat broiler.
- Marinate chicken.
- While chicken marinates, start barley.
- Make chicken dish.
- Finish barley dish.

1. Combine onion, garlic, chili powder, ground cumin, salt, and pepper in a bowl.

2. Remove visible fat from chicken, and poke several holes at varying intervals. Place in bowl, and spread chili mixture evenly over chicken on both sides. Let marinate 10 minutes, turning once.

3. Cover a baking tray with foil. Place chicken on the foil, and broil 4–5 inches from heat for 5 minutes; turn and broil 5 minutes. A meat thermometer should read 165°F.

4. Divide lettuce between two plates. Add tomato wedges to the lettuce. Slice chicken into strips and place on top of the lettuce.

5. Mix dressing and scallions together, and spoon over salad. Serve.

Preparation time: 25 ● Servings: 2

Calories 269 ● Calories from Fat 60 ● Total Fat 6.7 g ● Saturated Fat 1.2 g ● Monounsaturated Fat 2.0 g ● Cholesterol 109 mg ● Sodium 402 mg ● Carbohydrate 14.4 g ● Dietary Fiber 5.0 g ● Sugars 6.0 g ● Protein 39.3 g

Exchanges: 2 vegetable, 5 lean meat

Southwestern Barley Salad

1 cup water
1/3 cup pearl barley
1/2 cup frozen corn kernels
1 cup fresh diced onion
1/2 cup salsa ⚡
Salt

1. Pour water into medium saucepan, bring to a boil over high heat, and add barley. Cook 5 minutes.

2. Add corn and onion, bring back to a boil, cover, and continue to boil 5 minutes. Water will be absorbed and barley cooked through, but firm.

3. Add salsa and salt to taste and serve.

Preparation time: 15 minutes ● Servings: 2

Calories 201 ● Calories from Fat 10 ● Total Fat 1.1 g ● Saturated Fat 0.3 g ● Monounsaturated Fat 0.2 g ● Cholesterol 0 mg ● Sodium 142 mg ● Carbohydrate 44.2 g ● Dietary Fiber 8.3 g ● Sugars 7.9 g ● Protein 6.4 g

Exchanges: 2 1/2 starch, 1 vegetable

HELPFUL HINTS

■ Look for pearl barley.

■ Diced fresh onions can be found in the produce section of the supermarket.

■ Minced garlic can be found in jars in the produce or condiment sections of the supermarket.

SHOPPING LIST

Poultry
2 6-ounce boneless, skinless chicken breasts

Grocery
1 bottle chili powder
1 bottle ground cumin
1 package pearl barley
1 package frozen corn kernels
1 bottle salsa ⚡

Produce
1 large container fresh diced onion
1 bag washed ready-to-eat Romaine lettuce
1 medium tomato
1 small bunch scallions

Staple
Minced garlic
Reduced-fat oil and vinegar dressing ⚡
Salt
Black peppercorns

⚡ SHOP SMART!

Salsa (per 2 tablespoons): 10 calories, 2 g carbohydrate, 65 mg sodium [*Example*: Newman's Own All-Natural Bandito Salsa]

Reduced-fat vinaigrette or oil and vinegar dressing (per tablespoon): 11 calories, 1.0 g fat, 4 mg sodium

CHICKEN PIZZAIOLI WITH FENNEL AND BEAN SALAD

This chicken in a spicy tomato sauce is a real crowd pleaser.

The salad is made with fennel. Fennel has a large, pale green bulbous base with darker green stems and bright green feathery leaves. It's sometimes labeled anise in the market. Both the base and stems can be eaten raw or cooked. It has a very mild, sweet, licorice flavor. The fennel is very thinly sliced for this salad. Use a mandolin or the thin slicing blade on the food processor. It will take only a few minutes. Or slice the fennel by hand.

Chicken Pizzaioli

1 cup low-sodium pasta sauce ⚡
4 pitted black olives, cut in half
Several drops hot pepper sauce
Salt and freshly ground black pepper

Olive oil spray
1 teaspoon minced garlic
3/4 pound boneless, skinless chicken breast

COUNTDOWN
- Prepare ingredients.
- Start chicken.
- Make salad.
- Finish chicken.

1. Place pasta sauce and olives in a microwave-safe bowl. Cover and heat on high 1 minute. Or, place in a saucepan, and simmer 2–3 minutes or until heated through.
2. Add the hot pepper sauce and salt and pepper to taste.
3. Heat a nonstick skillet just large enough to hold chicken in one layer over medium-high heat. Spray with olive oil spray. Add the garlic and chicken. Brown on both sides, about 2 minutes.
4. Add sauce, lower heat to medium, cover with a lid, and cook 5 minutes. A meat thermometer should read 165°F. Remove from the skillet, and spoon sauce on top. Serve.

Preparation time: 15 minutes ● Servings: 2

Calories 337 ● Calories from Fat 96 ● Total Fat 10.7 g ● Saturated Fat 2.3 g ● Monounsaturated Fat 4.1 g ● Cholesterol 111 mg ● Sodium 304 mg ● Carbohydrate 19.7 g ● Dietary Fiber 3.7 g ● Sugars 11.4 g ● Protein 38.7 g

Exchanges: 1 1/2 starch, 5 lean meat

Fennel and Bean Salad

1 fennel bulb, thinly sliced (about 3 cups)
1 cup drained and rinsed cannellini or white navy beans
3 tablespoons reduced-fat Italian salad (oil and vinegar, not creamy) dressing ⚠
Salt and freshly ground black pepper

1. Cut the top stem and feathery leaves off the fennel. Reserve the fennel leaves.
2. Wash and slice the fennel bulb.
3. Place sliced fennel and beans in a bowl, and add dressing and salt and pepper to taste. Toss well.
4. Snip off about 1 tablespoon of the feathery leaves and sprinkle over salad. Serve.

Preparation time: 10 minutes ● Servings: 2

Calories 207 ● Calories from Fat 20 ● Total Fat 2.2 g ● Saturated Fat 0.3 g ● Monounsaturated Fat 0.5 g ● Cholesterol 1.5 mg ● Sodium 77 mg ● Carbohydrate 38.1 g ● Dietary Fiber 10.5 g ● Sugars 1.4 g ● Protein 11.4 g

Exchanges: 1 1/2 starch, 2 vegetable, 1 lean meat

HELPFUL HINTS:

■ Celery can be substituted for fennel.

■ The quickest way to chop the fennel leaves is to snip them with scissors.

■ Use a skillet just large enough to hold the chicken in one layer. If the skillet is too large, the sauce will run dry.

CHICKEN TOSTADAS AND CILANTRO TOMATOES

Crisp tortillas, smooth beans, hot flavors, and cool tomatoes make this a great, quick meal. *Tostado* is Spanish for "toasted," and a *tostada* is a flat tortilla that is toasted or deep fried. Tostadas are like little Mexican pizzas. They're usually served as an appetizer. The addition of chicken here makes this into a quick meal.

Chicken Tostadas

Olive oil spray
10 ounces boneless, skinless chicken breast cutlets (about 1/4-inch thick)
1 teaspoon ground cumin
Salt and freshly ground black pepper

4 6-inch corn tortillas
1/4 cup fat-free refried beans
2 tablespoons reduced-fat sour cream
1 cup shredded lettuce
1/4 cup fresh diced onion

COUNTDOWN
■ Sauté chicken.
■ Preheat broiler.
■ Prepare ingredients.
■ Make tomato salad.
■ Make tostadas.

1. Heat a medium skillet over medium-high heat. Spray with olive oil spray, and add chicken. Sauté 2 minutes; turn and sauté 2 more minutes. Sprinkle ground cumin and salt and pepper to taste over chicken. Transfer to a cutting board, and cut into 1/2-inch strips.

2. Preheat broiler. Line a baking tray with foil. Spray with olive oil spray.

3. Place tortillas on foil, and spray tortillas with olive oil spray.

4. Broil 2 minutes, remove from broiler, turn over, and broil 2 more minutes. The tortillas should be crisp. Divide between two dinner plates.

5. Spread refried beans over tortillas.

6. Spread sour cream over refried beans.

7. Divide chicken among the six tortillas.

8. Place lettuce on top of chicken. Sprinkle chopped onion over lettuce and serve.

Preparation time: 10 minutes ● Servings: 2

Calories 416 ● Calories from Fat 89 ● Total Fat 9.9 g ● Saturated Fat 2.5 g ● Monounsaturated Fat 3.8 g ● Cholesterol 96 mg ● Sodium 333 mg ● Carbohydrate 45.2 g ● Dietary Fiber 6.6 g ● Sugars 2.0 g ● Protein 37.2 g

Exchanges: 2 1/2 starch, 1 vegetable, 4 lean meat, 1/2 fat

Cilantro Tomatoes

1 cup fresh diced tomatoes
2 tablespoons chopped fresh cilantro
1 tablespoon olive oil
Salt and freshly ground black pepper

1. Mix tomatoes, cilantro, and olive oil together.
2. Sprinkle with salt and pepper to taste and serve.

Preparation time: 5 minutes ● Servings: 2

Calories 81 ● Calories from Fat 62 ● Total Fat 6.9 g ● Saturated Fat 1.0 g
● Monounsaturated Fat 5.0 g ● Cholesterol 0 mg ● Sodium 12 mg ●
Carbohydrate 4.8 g ● Dietary Fiber 1.2 g ● Sugars 2.9 g ● Protein 1.0 g

Exchanges: 1 vegetable, 1 1/2 fat

HELPFUL HINTS:

■ Diced fresh onions and tomatoes can be found in the produce section of the supermarket.

■ Tortillas can be made in a toaster oven instead of a broiler.

■ Shredded lettuce can be found in the produce section of the supermarket.

SHOPPING LIST

Poultry
10 ounces boneless, skinless chicken breast cutlets (about 1/4-inch thick)

Dairy
1 small carton reduced-fat sour cream

Grocery
1 package 6-inch corn tortillas
1 bottle ground cumin
1 can fat-free refried beans ❗

Produce
1 bag shredded lettuce
1 container fresh diced onion
1 container fresh diced tomatoes
1 bunch cilantro

Staples
Olive oil
Olive oil spray
Salt
Black peppercorns

❗ **SHOP SMART!**

Fat-free refried beans (per 1/2 cup): 100 calories, 0 g fat, 580 mg sodium [*Example*: El Paso Fat-Free Refried Beans]

CHICKEN AND GARLIC GREENS WITH SPICY SAUTÉED POTATOES

Get ready for a surprisingly different dinner with this grilled chicken topped with baby greens. In this recipe, baby greens, also known as field greens or mesclun, are sautéed with garlic to provide a colorful topping for the chicken. If you can't find the baby greens in the supermarket, you can use a soft lettuce, such as Bibb. Sautéing the greens for a minute enhances the flavor while retaining some of its crunch.

Potatoes usually take about 20 minutes to sauté. I microwave them first and then sauté them in the same skillet used for the chicken. Doing this saves you cooking and washing-up time.

Chicken and Garlic Greens

3/4 pound boneless, skinless chicken breast cutlets (about 1/4-inch thick)

1/4 cup balsamic vinegar (discarded in marinade)

Olive oil spray

Salt and freshly ground black pepper

2 teaspoons olive oil

2 teaspoons minced garlic

4 cups washed ready-to-eat mesclun or field greens (4 ounces)

COUNTDOWN

- Marinate chicken.
- Prepare remaining ingredients.
- Microwave potatoes.
- Sauté chicken.
- Sauté potatoes using same skillet as chicken.

1. Remove visible fat from chicken. Add balsamic vinegar to a self-sealing plastic bag or bowl. Add chicken. Let stand 5 minutes, turning once during that time.

2. Heat a nonstick skillet over medium-high heat and spray with olive oil spray. Remove chicken from bag, and discard marinade. Place chicken in skillet, and sauté 3 minutes; turn and sauté 2 minutes. A meat thermometer should read 165°F. Sprinkle with salt and pepper to taste. Transfer to a plate.

3. Add oil and garlic to the skillet. Sauté 30 seconds. Add greens and toss in pan, about 2 minutes. Salad should be warm but remain firm. Add salt and pepper to taste, and spoon over chicken. Serve.

Preparation time: 15 minutes ● Servings: 2

Calories 273 ● Calories from Fat 96 ● Total Fat 10.7 g ● Saturated Fat 1.8 g ● Monounsaturated Fat 5.6 g ● Cholesterol 108 mg ● Sodium 211 mg ● Carbohydrate 6.0 g ● Dietary Fiber 2.2 g ● Sugars 1.7 g ● Protein 37.7 g

Exchanges: 1 vegetable, 5 lean meat, 1/2 fat

Spicy Sautéed Potatoes

1 pound red potatoes
1 tablespoon olive oil
1/8 teaspoon cayenne pepper
Salt

1. Wash potatoes (do not peel), and cut into 1-inch pieces. Place in a bowl, and microwave on high 4 minutes.

2. Meanwhile, add oil and cayenne pepper to the same skillet used for the chicken, after the greens have been removed.

3. Add the microwaved potatoes, and toss in the skillet 5 minutes. Add salt to taste and serve.

Preparation time: 10 minutes ● Servings: 2

Calories 219 ● Calories from Fat 64 ● Total Fat 7.1 g ● Saturated Fat 1.0 g ● Monounsaturated Fat 4.9 g ● Cholesterol 0 mg ● Sodium 14 mg ● Carbohydrate 36.2 g ● Dietary Fiber 3.9 g ● Sugars 2.3 g ● Protein 4.3 g

Exchanges: 2 1/2 starch, 1 fat

SHOPPING LIST

Poultry
3/4 pound boneless, skinless chicken breast cutlets

Grocery
1 bottle cayenne pepper

Produce
1 bag washed ready-to-eat mesclun or field greens
1 pound red potatoes

Staples
Olive oil
Olive oil spray
Balsamic vinegar
Minced garlic
Salt
Black peppercorns

HELPFUL HINTS:

■ Any type of waxy potato, such as yellow or creamers, can be used.

■ Use a self-sealing plastic bag for marinating. To turn meat over, simply flip over the bag. This saves you from having to wash a bowl.

■ The heat is up to you. Add more cayenne if you like your potatoes really hot.

CHICKEN AND SHIITAKE YAKITORI

Yakitori are Japanese grilled chicken kabobs made with a sweet Japanese barbecue sauce. The secret to quick and even kabob cooking is to leave a little space on the skewer between each piece of chicken. This allows the chicken to cook through on all sides.

Chicken and Shiitake Yakitori (Japanese Grilled Chicken Skewers)

Olive oil spray

2 tablespoons reduced-sodium teriyaki sauce 🔋

4 tablespoons rice wine vinegar

2 tablespoons honey

1/4 pound shiitake mushrooms (about 1 2/3 cups)

3/4 pound boneless, skinless chicken breast, cut into 1-inch cubes

1 red bell pepper, cut into 2-inch pieces (about 1 1/2 cups)

4 skewers

COUNTDOWN

- Make sauce and marinate chicken and mushrooms.
- Make rice and set aside.
- Heat a stove-top grill.
- Skewer and cook kabobs.

1. Heat a stove-top grill over high heat. Spray with olive oil spray.

2. Mix teriyaki sauce, rice wine vinegar, and honey in a small saucepan. Add mushrooms, chicken, and bell pepper, and marinate 5 minutes while rice is started. Remove mushrooms, chicken, and pepper from sauce, making sure to reserve sauce.

3. Place chicken, mushroom, and red pepper on skewers, alternating the ingredients until the skewers are full. Leave at least 1/4-inch space between ingredients.

4. Place on stove-top grill and cook 5 minutes; turn and cook 5 more minutes.

5. Bring reserved sauce to a boil, and cook 3 minutes. Spoon over cooked kabobs and serve.

Preparation time: 20 minutes ● Servings: 2

Calories 347 ● Calories from Fat 63 ● Total Fat 7.1 g ● Saturated Fat 1.3 g ● Monounsaturated Fat 2.8 g ● Cholesterol 108 mg ● Sodium 547 mg ● Carbohydrate 29.5 g ● Dietary Fiber 2.9 g ● Sugars 24.6 g ● Protein 40.2 g

Exchanges: 1 carbohydrate, 2 vegetable, 5 lean meat

Sesame Rice

1 package microwaveable brown rice (1 1/2 cup used)
1 tablespoon sesame oil
Salt and freshly ground black pepper

1. Microwave rice according to package instructions.
2. Measure 1 1/2 cups cooked rice. Reserve remaining rice for another meal.
3. Add sesame oil and salt and pepper to taste. Serve.

Preparation time: 3 minutes ● Servings: 2

Calories 240 ● Calories from Fat 84 ● Total Fat 9.4 g ● Saturated Fat 1.3 g ● Monounsaturated Fat 3.5 g ● Cholesterol 0 mg ● Sodium 11 mg ● Carbohydrate 29.3 g ● Dietary Fiber 1.5 g ● Sugars 0 g ● Protein 3.8 g

Exchanges: 2 starch, 2 fat

HELPFUL HINTS:

■ Any type of mushrooms can be used.

■ If using wooden skewers, soak them in water for about 30 minutes before use.

■ The skewers can also be cooked under a broiler or an outdoor grill.

SHOPPING LIST

Poultry
3/4 pound boneless, skinless chicken breast

Grocery
1 small bottle reduced-sodium teriyaki sauce ⚠
1 small bottle rice wine vinegar
1 small bottle honey
1 package microwaveable brown rice
1 bottle sesame oil

Produce
1/4 pound shiitake mushrooms
1 red bell pepper

Staples
Olive oil spray
Salt
Black peppercorns

⚠ SHOP SMART!

Reduced-sodium teriyaki sauce (per tablespoon): 8 calories, 1.5 g carbohydrate, 168 mg sodium

CHICKEN AND WALNUTS IN LETTUCE PUFFS WITH CHINESE RICE

This stir-fry dish is one of my favorites. Crisp, cool lettuce topped with warm chicken and vegetables combine to create a sensational taste and texture combination.

This is a 20-minute meal. As with most Chinese recipes, there are several ingredients to be prepared, but the actual cooking time is only about 4–5 minutes.

Chicken and Walnuts in Lettuce Puffs

1/2 pound boneless, skinless chicken breast, cut into 1/2-inch pieces

1 1/2 tablespoons oyster sauce 🔲

3 teaspoons sesame oil, divided

1 teaspoon minced garlic

1/2 cup shiitake mushrooms, diced

1/2 cup canned sliced water chestnuts, drained (2 1/2 ounces)

1/4 cup unsalted walnut pieces

8 small iceberg lettuce cups (inner leaves from lettuce that curve into a cup)

COUNTDOWN

- Prepare walnuts and chicken.
- While chicken marinates, prepare all other ingredients.
- Start rice.
- Stir-fry the dish.

1. Place chicken in a bowl with oyster sauce, and let stand 5 minutes.
2. Heat wok over high heat. Add 1 teaspoon sesame oil. Add chicken, and stir-fry for 1 minute.
3. Add garlic, mushrooms, and water chestnuts. Stir-fry 2 minutes.
4. Add remaining 2 teaspoons sesame oil. Cook a few seconds to heat through. Add walnuts, and toss to coat. Remove from heat.
5. To serve, divide 4 lettuce cups between two dinner plates. Spoon some of chicken mixture into each lettuce cup, wrap, and eat.

Preparation time: 10 minutes ● Servings: 2

Calories 370 ● Calories from Fat 179 ● Total Fat 19.9 g ● Saturated Fat 2.6 g ● Monounsaturated Fat 5.0 g ● Cholesterol 72 mg ● Sodium 513 mg ● Carbohydrate 20.0 g ● Dietary Fiber 3.3 g ● Sugars 1.5 g ● Protein 29.4 g

Exchanges: 1 1/2 carbohydrate, 4 lean meat, 2 fats

Chinese Rice

1/2 cup long-grain white rice
3/4 cup water
3 scallions, sliced (1/2 cup)
1 teaspoon sesame oil
Salt and freshly ground black pepper

1. Place rice in a medium saucepan. Add water. Cover and bring to a boil over high heat.
2. Stir, lower heat to medium, cover, and continue to boil, about 10 minutes.
3. Remove cover. Stir to make sure no rice sticks to the bottom of the pan. If rice is still very moist, simmer uncovered until only a few drops of moisture remain.
4. Add scallions, oil, and salt and pepper to taste. Remove from heat. Cover and let stand 5 minutes. Loosen rice by tossing the rice with a fork to separate the grains before serving. Serve.

Preparation time: 20 minutes ● Servings: 2

Calories 197 ● Calories from Fat 24 ● Total Fat 2.6 g ● Saturated Fat 0.4 g ● Monounsaturated Fat 1.0 g ● Cholesterol 0 mg ● Sodium 6 mg ● Carbohydrate 38.8 g ● Dietary Fiber 1.3 g ● Sugars 0.6 g ● Protein 3.8 g

Exchanges: 2 1/2 starch

SHOPPING LIST

Poultry
8 ounces boneless, skinless chicken breast

Grocery
1 bottle oyster sauce **!**
1 small container unsalted walnuts
1 bottle sesame oil
1 can sliced canned water chestnuts
1 package long-grain white rice

Produce
1 package shiitake mushrooms
1 small head iceberg lettuce
1 bunch scallions

Staples
Minced garlic
Salt
Black peppercorns

! SHOP SMART!

Oyster sauce (per tablespoon):
9 calories, 492 mg sodium

HELPFUL HINTS:

■ Use toasted sesame oil if available in your market. It gives a smoky flavor.

■ Dry sherry can be substituted for the Chinese rice wine.

CHINESE SALAD WITH ASIAN DRESSING

This is a simple one-dish meal made with shiitake mushrooms, chicken, cashews, and an Asian dressing. It can be served warm or at room temperature. I've provided substitutions for some of the Chinese ingredients, so you can make this salad with ingredients you have on hand, if you prefer.

Chinese Salad with Asian Dressing

2 teaspoons reduced-sodium soy sauce

3 tablespoons Chinese rice vinegar

1 tablespoon toasted sesame oil, divided

1/4 pound steamed or dried Chinese noodles (about 1/2 cup)

3/4 pound boneless, skinless chicken breast, cut into 1/2-inch pieces

3 teaspoons minced garlic

1 red bell pepper, sliced (about 1 1/2 cups)

1 cup sliced shiitake or Portobello mushrooms

Salt and freshly ground black pepper

3 cups washed ready-to-eat Romaine lettuce

2 scallions, sliced (about 1/3 cup)

2 tablespoons unsalted cashew nuts

COUNTDOWN

- Place water for Chinese noodles on to boil.
- Mix sauce.
- Boil noodles.
- Make salad.

1. Place a medium saucepan filled with water on to boil over high heat.

2. Mix the soy sauce, vinegar, and 1/2 tablespoon sesame oil together. Set aside.

3. When water comes to a boil, add the noodles. Boil 2 minutes, and drain in a colander. Run cold water through them. Set aside.

4. Heat the remaining 1/2 tablespoon sesame oil in a wok or nonstick skillet over high heat. Add the chicken, and stir-fry 2 minutes. Add garlic, red pepper, and mushrooms. Stir-fry 2 minutes. Add the soy sauce mixture, and stir-fry 1 minute. Remove wok from the heat, and add the noodles. Add salt and pepper to taste. Toss well.

5. Divide lettuce leaves between two dinner plates. Spoon noodle and meat mixture over lettuce. Sprinkle sliced scallion and cashews on top. Serve.

Preparation time: 10 minutes ● Servings: 2

Calories 526 ● Calories from Fat 158 ● Total Fat 17.6 g ● Saturated Fat 3.1 g ● Monounsaturated Fat 6.4 g ● Cholesterol 144 mg ● Sodium 492 mg ● Carbohydrate 44.9 g ● Dietary Fiber 6.2 g ● Sugars 7.7 g ● Protein 47.1 g

Exchanges: 2 starch, 2 vegetable, 5 lean meat, 2 fat

HELPFUL HINTS:

■ White vinegar diluted with a little water can be used instead of rice vinegar.

■ Any variety of cooked chicken—strips, pieces, roasted, or rotisserie—can be used.

■ Sesame oil lends a nutty flavor. Toasted sesame oil can be found in most supermarkets. I prefer its more intense sesame flavor.

■ Regular sesame oil or canola oil can be used instead of toasted sesame oil.

■ Steamed Chinese noodles can be found in the refrigerated section of the produce department. Dried Chinese noodles or angel hair pasta can be used instead.

■ Any sliced mushrooms can be used instead of shiitake.

■ Minced garlic can be found in jars in the produce section of the market.

■ Walnuts can be used instead of cashew nuts.

■ A quick way to slice scallions is to snip them with scissors.

SHOPPING LIST

Poultry
3/4 pound boneless, skinless chicken breast

Grocery
1 bottle reduced-sodium soy sauce
1 bottle Chinese rice vinegar
1 package steamed or dried Chinese noodles
1 bottle toasted sesame oil
1 package unsalted cashew nuts

Produce
1 red bell pepper
1 container shiitake or Portobello mushrooms
1 bag washed ready-to-eat Romaine lettuce
1 bunch scallions

Staples
Minced garlic
Salt
Black peppercorns

COQ AU VIN (CHICKEN STEWED IN RED WINE) WITH BROWN RICE

French peasants cooked with whatever they had on hand. *Coq au vin* was made with an old rooster, leftover red wine, onions, carrots, and celery. It would be cooked for hours. This is a quick version of the celebrated French dish.

Coq au Vin (Chicken Stewed in Red Wine)

2 chicken breasts on the bone (3/4 pound each), skin and wing removed
2 teaspoons olive oil
1/2 cup sliced carrot
1 cup fresh diced celery
1 tablespoon flour
1 medium tomato, cut into 6 segments
1 teaspoon dried thyme
2 teaspoons minced garlic
1 ounce lean ham (about 1/3 cup)
1 cup red burgundy or other red wine
1/2 cup fat-free, low-sodium chicken broth
1/4 pound sliced button mushrooms (about 1 2/3 cups)
Salt and freshly ground black pepper

COUNTDOWN

■ Prepare chicken ingredients.
■ Start chicken.
■ While chicken cooks, make rice.
■ Finish chicken.

1. Cut chicken into 4 pieces, if it wasn't cut at the market.
2. Heat olive oil in nonstick skillet over high heat. Add the chicken, and brown on both sides, about 5 minutes.
3. Add the carrot and celery. Sauté with the chicken 2–3 minutes or until vegetables start to shrivel. Sprinkle flour over vegetables, and stir until absorbed by vegetables.
4. Add the tomato, thyme, garlic, ham, red wine, and chicken broth. Bring to a simmer. Lower heat to medium, cover with foil and then with a lid, and simmer 15 minutes.
5. Add the mushrooms, and continue to cook 5 minutes. Add salt and pepper to taste. Serve.

Preparation time: 30 minutes ● Servings: 2

Calories 360 ● Calories from Fat 90 ● Total Fat 10.0 g ● Saturated Fat 1.8 g ● Monounsaturated Fat 4.8 g ● Cholesterol 115 mg ● Sodium 564 mg ● Carbohydrate 16.6 g ● Dietary Fiber 3.9 g ● Sugars 5.0 g ● Protein 43.7 g

Exchanges: 3 vegetable, 5 lean meat, 1/2 fat, 1/2 alcohol

Brown Rice

1 package microwaveable brown rice (1 1/2 cups cooked)
2 teaspoons olive oil
Salt and freshly ground black pepper

1. Cook brown rice according to package instructions in the microwave. Measure 1 1/2 cups cooked rice, and reserve remaining rice for another meal.
2. Add oil, salt, and pepper to taste. Toss well. Serve with chicken.

Preparation time: 5 minutes ● Servings: 2

Calories 209 ● Calories from Fat 43 ● Total Fat 4.8 g ● Saturated Fat 0.7 g ● Monounsaturated Fat 3.4 g ● Cholesterol 0 mg ● Sodium 2 mg ● Carbohydrate 37.0 g ● Dietary Fiber 0.6 g ● Sugars 0.1 g ● Protein 3.3 g

Exchanges: 2 1/2 starch, 1/2 fat

HELPFUL HINTS:

■ Ask the butcher to cut each chicken breast with the bone into four pieces.

■ Fresh diced celery can be found in the produce section of the supermarket.

■ Minced garlic can be found in jars in the produce or condiment sections of the supermarket.

■ Cover the chicken, vegetables, and sauce with foil and then with a lid. This will keep the chicken from drying out and the sauce from evaporating.

SHOPPING LIST

Poultry
2 3/4-pound chicken breasts on the bone

Deli
1 ounce lean ham *!*

Grocery
1 bottle dried thyme
1 bottle red burgundy or other red wine
1 package microwaveable brown rice

Produce
1 package sliced carrots
1 container fresh diced celery
1 medium tomato
1/4 pound sliced button mushrooms

Staples
Olive oil
Minced garlic
Flour
Fat-free, low-sodium chicken broth
Salt
Black peppercorns

! SHOP SMART!

Lean ham (per ounce): 30 calories, 0.7 g fat, 0.2 g saturated fat, 301 mg sodium

COUNTRY MUSHROOM AND SAUSAGE SOUP WITH ONION-GARLIC CROSTINI

This soup supper is made to order for a busy weeknight. Most people think that for a soup to be good, it has to cook for hours. I love soup suppers and decided to create this tomato-based mushroom and sausage soup that takes only 20 minutes to make.

Onion-garlic crostini or "little toasts" are a great accompaniment for this dinner.

Country Mushroom and Sausage Soup

2 teaspoons olive oil
1 pound sliced button mushrooms
1 4-ounce turkey sausage, sliced 🔳
1 cup fat-free, low-sodium pasta sauce 🔳

1 cup cannellini beans, rinsed and drained
1 cup fat-free, low-sodium chicken broth
1 cup water

COUNTDOWN

■ Start soup.
■ While soup cooks, prepare crostini.

1. Heat olive oil in a large saucepan over medium-high heat. Add the mushrooms and sausage. Sauté 2 minutes, stirring to brown sausage.

2. Add the pasta sauce, beans, broth, and water. Bring to a simmer, cover with a lid, and simmer 15 minutes. Divide between two soup bowls and serve.

Preparation time: 20 minutes ● Servings: 2

Calories 447 ● Calories from Fat 125 ● Total Fat 13.8 g ● Saturated Fat 2.9 g ● Monounsaturated Fat 5.6 g ● Cholesterol 45 mg ● Sodium 676 mg ● Carbohydrate 53.6 g ● Dietary Fiber 12.1 g ● Sugars 11.7 g ● Protein 31.3 g

Exchanges: 2 1/2 starch, 2 vegetable, 3 lean meat, 1 1/2 fat

Onion-Garlic Crostini

1 cup fresh diced red onion
1 teaspoon minced garlic
1 teaspoon olive oil
1 teaspoon sugar
2 large slices multigrain country bread
Olive oil spray

Microwave method
1. Place onion and garlic in a microwave-safe bowl. Microwave on high 2 minutes. Remove and stir in olive oil and sugar.

Stove-top method
1. Heat a medium nonstick skillet over medium heat, and add olive oil. Add onion and garlic, and sauté, without burning, for 10 minutes. Add sugar, and sauté another 5 minutes.

2. Spray bread with olive oil spray and toast in toaster oven or under broiler until golden, about 1 minute. Spoon onion mixture over bread, and serve with soup.

Preparation time: 5 minutes for microwave method ● Servings: 2

Calories 138 ● Calories from Fat 44 ● Total Fat 4.9 g ● Saturated Fat 0.8 g ● Monounsaturated Fat 2.9 g ● Cholesterol 0 mg ● Sodium 115 mg ● Carbohydrate 20.1g ● Dietary Fiber 3.0 g ● Sugars 6.2 g ● Protein 4.3 g

Exchanges: 1 starch, 1 vegetable, 1/2 fat

HELPFUL HINTS:

■ Navy beans or red kidney beans can be used instead of cannellini beans.

■ Any leftover whole-grain bread can be used for the crostini.

■ Diced fresh onions can be found in the produce section of the supermarket.

■ Minced garlic can be found in jars in the produce or condiment sections of the supermarket.

SHOPPING LIST

Poultry
1 package turkey sausage ⚠

Grocery
1 bottle fat-free, low-sodium pasta sauce ⚠
1 can cannellini beans
1 loaf multigrain country bread

Produce
1 pound sliced button mushrooms
1 container fresh diced red onion

Staples
Olive oil
Olive oil spray
Minced garlic
Sugar
Fat-free, low-sodium chicken broth

⚠ SHOP SMART!

Turkey sausage (per ounce): 44 calories, 2.20 g fat, 0.6 saturated fat, 168 mg sodium

Low-sodium pasta sauce (per 1/2 cup): 112 calories, 3.5 g fat, 17.7 g carbohydrate, 39 mg sodium

CRISPY CHICKEN WITH RATATOUILLE (SAUTÉED PROVENÇAL VEGETABLES)

Ratatouille is a tasty blend of Provençal vegetables and is made by slowly simmering eggplant, zucchini, onion, garlic, and tomatoes in olive oil. Using bottled pasta sauce, this quick version captures the flavors of Provence without the lengthy cooking time. Coating the chicken with coarse cornmeal gives it a crisp, flavorful crust without having to deep-fry it.

Crispy Chicken

1/4 cup coarse cornmeal
Salt and freshly ground black pepper
1 egg white

3/4 pound chicken breast cutlets (about 1/4-inch thick)
1 tablespoon olive oil

COUNTDOWN

■ Start ratatouille.
■ Make chicken.

1. Season cornmeal with salt and pepper to taste.
2. Lightly beat egg white with a fork. Dip chicken into egg white and then cornmeal, making sure both sides are well coated.
3. Heat olive oil in a nonstick skillet over medium-high heat. Add chicken, and sauté 2 minutes; turn and sauté 2 more minutes. A meat thermometer should read 165°F. Divide between two dinner plates and serve.

Preparation time: 10 minutes ● Servings: 2

Calories 333 ● Calories from Fat 104 ● Total Fat 11.5 g ● Saturated Fat 1.9 g ● Monounsaturated Fat 6.3 g ● Cholesterol 108 mg ● Sodium 227 mg ● Carbohydrate 15.9 g ● Dietary Fiber 0.8 g ● Sugars 0.5 g ● Protein 39.4 g

Exchanges: 1 starch, 5 lean meat, 1 fat

Ratatouille (Sautéed Provençal Vegetables)

1/2 pound eggplant, washed, unpeeled, and sliced (about 2 1/2 cups)
1/2 pound zucchini, washed and sliced (about 2 cups)
2 cups sliced button mushrooms
1 1/2 cups low-sodium pasta sauce ❗
Salt and freshly ground black pepper

1. If eggplant slices are large, cut them in half. Add eggplant, zucchini, mushrooms, and pasta sauce to a medium saucepan.

2. Bring to a simmer over medium heat. Lower heat and cover. Simmer 15 minutes.

3. Vegetables should be cooked through but a little firm. Add salt and pepper to taste and serve.

Preparation time: 20 minutes ● Servings: 2

Calories 226 ● Calories from Fat 52 ● Total Fat 5.8 g ● Saturated Fat 1.5 g ● Monounsaturated Fat 1.2 g ● Cholesterol 4 mg ● Sodium 75 mg ● Carbohydrate 38.5 g ● Dietary Fiber 10.4 g ● Sugars 21.4 g ● Protein 8.0 g

Exchanges: 2 starch, 1 vegetable, 1 fat

HELPFUL HINTS:

■ Any type of cornmeal can be used.

■ Boneless, skinless chicken breasts can be used instead of chicken cutlets. Flatten them to about 1/4-inch thick.

SHOPPING LIST

Poultry
3/4 pound chicken breast cutlets
   (1/4-inch thick)

Grocery
1 package coarse cornmeal
1 bottle low-sodium pasta sauce ❗

Produce
1/2 pound eggplant
1/2 pound zucchini
1 container sliced button mushrooms

Staples
Egg
Olive oil
Salt
Black peppercorns

❗ SHOP SMART!

Low-sodium pasta sauce (per 1/2 cup): 112 calories, 3.5 g fat, 17.7 g carbohydrate, 39 mg sodium

CURRIED CHICKEN POT PIE

Pot pies are warm and inviting. The curry powder in the sauce gives this pie an intriguing flavor. Using prepared ingredients from the supermarket, you can put this one-pot meal together in only 30 minutes. Using seasoned bread crumbs over the ingredients instead of a pie crust shortens the cooking time even further.

Curried Chicken Pot Pie

1 tablespoon canola oil

3/4 pound chicken cutlets (1/4-inch thick), cut into 1/2-inch cubes

1/2 tablespoon mild curry powder

1 cup fresh diced onion

1 cup fresh diced green bell pepper

1/4 pound sliced baby bello mushrooms (about 1 1/2 cups)

2 tablespoons flour

1 cup fat-free low-sodium chicken broth

1 cup frozen peas

Salt and freshly ground black pepper

1 cup plain bread crumbs

2 tablespoons grated Parmesan cheese

COUNTDOWN

- Preheat oven to 400°F.
- Prepare pie ingredients.
- Make pie.

1. Preheat oven to 400°F. Heat the oil in a large nonstick skillet over medium-high heat. Add the chicken, and sauté 2 minutes.

2. Add curry powder, onion, green bell pepper, and mushrooms. Sauté 5 minutes.

3. Add the flour to the mixture, stir to blend, and add the chicken broth. Simmer to thicken, about 1 minute. Mix the peas into the sauce. Add salt and pepper to taste.

4. Spoon into a deep ovenproof pie dish or a soufflé dish about 6 inches in diameter.

5. Sprinkle bread crumbs and Parmesan cheese over the top.

6. Bake for 20 minutes. Remove from oven and serve.

Preparation time: 30 minutes ● Servings: 2

Calories 635 ● Calories from Fat 147 ● Total Fat 16.4 g ● Saturated Fat 3.2 g ● Monounsaturated Fat 6.7 g ● Cholesterol 112 mg ● Sodium 759 mg ● Carbohydrate 68.6 g ● Dietary Fiber 9.4 g ● Sugars 12.5 g ● Protein 53.3 g

Exchanges: 3 1/2 starch, 2 vegetable, 6 lean meat, 1/2 fat

HELPFUL HINTS:

- Diced fresh onions and green bell pepper can be found in the produce section of the supermarket.

- Any type of sliced mushrooms can be used.

SHOPPING LIST

Poultry
3/4 pound chicken cutlets
    (1/4-inch thick)

Dairy
1 small container best-quality grated
    Parmesan cheese

Grocery
1 bottle mild curry powder
1 package frozen peas
1 container plain bread crumbs

Produce
1/4 pound sliced baby bello
    mushrooms
1 container fresh diced onion
1 container fresh green bell pepper

Staples
Canola oil
Flour
Fat-free low-sodium chicken broth
Salt
Black peppercorns

DIJON CHICKEN WITH VEGETABLE QUINOA

This sauce—made with Dijon mustard and dry vermouth—flavors thin-sliced chicken cutlets. Quinoa is an ancient grain that is high in protein and a good source of fiber.

Dijon Chicken

Olive oil spray
3/4 pound boneless, skinless thin-sliced chicken cutlet
1/2 cup dry vermouth (or white wine)

3 tablespoons Dijon mustard
4 tablespoons fat-free half and half
Salt and freshly ground black pepper

COUNTDOWN

■ Place water for quinoa on to boil.
■ Make chicken.
■ Finish quinoa.

1. Heat a nonstick skillet over medium-high heat, and spray with olive oil spray. Brown chicken 2 minutes; turn and brown 2 more minutes.

2. Transfer chicken to two dinner plates. A meat thermometer should read 165°F.

3. Add vermouth to the skillet. Boil for 30 seconds, add mustard, and stir to blend to a smooth sauce, about 30 seconds.

4. Remove from heat. Add half and half and salt and pepper to taste. Spoon sauce over chicken and serve.

Preparation time: 10 minutes ● Servings: 2

Calories 281 ● Calories from Fat 64 ● Total Fat 7.1 g ● Saturated Fat 1.5 g ● Monounsaturated Fat 3.0 g ● Cholesterol 109 mg ● Sodium 499 mg ● Carbohydrate 4.4 g ● Dietary Fiber 0.8 g ● Sugars 1.6 g ● Protein 37.9 g

Exchanges: 5 lean meat, 1/2 alcohol

Vegetable Quinoa

3/4 cup quinoa
1/2 pound broccoli florets, cut in half (about 4 cups)
2 teaspoons olive oil
Salt and freshly ground black pepper

1. Bring a large saucepan filled with water to a boil over high heat.

2. Add the quinoa. Boil 5 minutes.

3. Add broccoli, bring back to a boil, and continue to boil 3 minutes.

4. Drain, leaving 2 tablespoons water in the saucepan.

5. Add olive oil and salt and pepper to taste to the saucepan. Return quinoa and broccoli, and toss well. Serve with chicken.

Preparation time: 15 minutes ● Servings: 2

Calories 307 ● Calories from Fat 79 ● Total Fat 8.8 g ● Saturated Fat 1.1 g ● Monounsaturated Fat 4.3 g ● Cholesterol 0 mg ● Sodium 33 mg ● Carbohydrate 46.9 g ● Dietary Fiber 4.5 g ● Sugars 0 g ● Protein 12.4 g

Exchanges: 2 1/2 starch, 2 vegetable, 1 1/2 fat

SHOPPING LIST

Poultry
3/4 pound boneless, skinless thin-sliced chicken cutlet

Dairy
1 small carton fat-free half and half

Grocery
1 small bottle dry vermouth
1 bottle Dijon mustard
1 package quinoa

Produce
1/2 pound broccoli florets

Staples
Olive oil
Olive oil spray
Salt
Black peppercorns

HELPFUL HINTS:

■ Any type of green vegetable can be used with the quinoa, such as trimmed green beans or zucchini.

■ If thin chicken cutlets are not available, use boneless, skinless chicken breasts and cut in half horizontally to make 1/4-inch cutlets.

■ Fat-free, low-sodium chicken broth can be used instead of vermouth.

GRILLED CHICKEN WRAPS AND PARMESAN CORN

Grilled chicken thighs and onion fill these tasty dinner wraps. Corn on the cob with a Parmesan coating takes only minutes to make in the microwave oven.

Grilled Chicken Wraps

3/4 pound boneless, skinless chicken thighs
Salt and freshly ground black pepper
2 1/4-inch onion slices (about 1/2 cup)
1/4 cup low-sugar, low-sodium barbecue sauce ⚡

2 8-inch whole-wheat flour tortillas
1/2 cup shredded lettuce
1/2 cup fresh diced tomatoes

COUNTDOWN

- Heat a stove-top grill.
- Place chicken, onion, and corn on the grill.
- Prepare tomatoes and lettuce.
- When chicken and onion are ready, make wraps.
- Microwave corn.

1. Preheat a stove-top grill.
2. Remove visible fat from chicken, and season with salt and pepper to taste.
3. Place chicken and onion slices on the grill. Cook 5 minutes. Turn chicken and onions over, and grill 3 minutes. Spoon barbecue sauce over chicken and onion, and grill 2 minutes. A meat thermometer should reach 165°F. Transfer to a plate. Using two forks, shred the chicken. Separate the onions into rings.
4. Meanwhile, wrap the tortillas in foil and add to the grill for 3 minutes to warm through. Fill each tortilla with some of the chicken and onions, and roll into a wrap.
5. Divide lettuce between two plates, and top with diced tomatoes. Serve.

Preparation time: 20 minutes ● Servings: 2

Calories 363 ● Calories from Fat 74 ● Total Fat 8.2 g ● Saturated Fat 2.2 g ● Monounsaturated Fat 2.1 g ● Cholesterol 138 mg ● Sodium 335 mg ● Carbohydrate 32.5 g ● Dietary Fiber 3.5 g ● Sugars 11.7 g ● Protein 37.6 g

Exchanges: 1 1/2 starch, 1 vegetable, 1/2 carbohydrate, 4 lean meat

Parmesan Corn

2 medium ears of corn, shucked
2 teaspoons canola oil
1 tablespoon best-quality grated Parmesan cheese
Salt and freshly ground black pepper

1. Shuck corn, and wrap each ear in a damp paper towel.

2. Place the ears on a dinner plate, and microwave on high 2 minutes. Turn corn over and microwave on high 1 1/2 minutes.

3. Remove paper towel, and rub corn with oil. Sprinkle Parmesan cheese over corn, add salt and pepper to taste, and serve.

Preparation time: 5 minutes ● Servings: 2

Calories 139 ● Calories from Fat 59 ● Total Fat 6.6 g ● Saturated Fat 1.1 g ● Monounsaturated Fat 3.5 g ● Cholesterol 2 mg ● Sodium 53 mg ● Carbohydrate 19.1 g ● Dietary Fiber 2.0 g ● Sugars 6.4 g ● Protein 4.3 g

Exchanges: 1 starch, 1 1/2 fat

HELPFUL HINTS:

■ Diced fresh tomatoes can be found in the produce section of the supermarket.

■ Look for Parmigiano-Reggiano cheese.

■ Chicken and onions can be made in a skillet if a stove-top grill is not available.

SHOPPING LIST

Poultry
3/4 pound boneless, skinless chicken thighs

Dairy
1 small container best-quality grated Parmesan cheese

Grocery
1 bottle low-sugar, low-sodium barbecue sauce ❗
1 package 8-inch whole-wheat tortillas

Produce
1 container fresh diced tomatoes
1 bag shredded lettuce
2 medium ears corn

Staples
Onion
Canola oil
Salt
Black peppercorns

❗ SHOP SMART!

Low-sugar, low-sodium barbecue sauce (per tablespoon): 26 calories, 6.3 g carbohydrate, 23 mg sodium

HAWAIIAN CHICKEN WITH PINEAPPLE SALAD

Chicken with a pineapple-laced barbecue sauce served with a tropical salad are an attractive combination in this easy-to-serve dinner. A barbecue sauce that contains sugar can burn and blacken the food. The secret is to use the sauce as a glaze, painting the food during the last few minutes of cooking.

Hawaiian Chicken

1/4 cup low-sodium pasta sauce **!**

2 tablespoons pineapple juice (from pineapple cubes container)

2 teaspoons Dijon mustard

2 teaspoons sugar

Olive oil spray

2 6-ounce boneless, skinless chicken breast cutlets (1/4-inch thick)

Salt and freshly ground black pepper

2 whole-wheat rolls (2 ounces each)

COUNTDOWN

■ Prepare chicken.
■ Make salad.

1. Mix pasta sauce, pineapple juice, mustard, and sugar together to make a sauce.

2. Heat a nonstick skillet over medium-high heat, and spray with olive oil spray. Sear chicken 3 minutes; turn and sear second side 3 minutes. Add salt and pepper to taste to the cooked side. A meat thermometer should read 165°F.

3. Remove from heat, and spoon sauce over chicken. Divide between two dinner plates.

4. Cut rolls open, spray with olive oil spray, and toast. Serve chicken with rolls on the side.

Preparation time: 10 minutes ● Servings: 2

Calories 410 ● Calories from Fat 85 ● Total Fat 9.5 g ● Saturated Fat 1.9 g ● Monounsaturated Fat 3.3 g ● Cholesterol 109 mg ● Sodium 535 mg ● Carbohydrate 39.3 g ● Dietary Fiber 5.3 g ● Sugars 11.8 g ● Protein 41.8 g

Exchanges: 2 1/2 starch, 5 lean meat

Pineapple Salad

1 cup fresh pineapple cubes (if large, cut in half)
4 cups washed ready-to-eat Romaine lettuce
2 tablespoons bottled reduced-fat oil and vinegar dressing ❗
8 or 9 macadamia nuts

1. Place pineapple cubes and lettuce in a salad bowl. Add dressing. Toss well. Sprinkle the top with macadamia nuts. Serve with the chicken.

Preparation time: 5 minutes ● Servings: 2

Calories 142 ● Calories from Fat 87 ● Total Fat 9.7 g ● Saturated Fat 1.4 g ● Monounsaturated Fat 6.7 g ● Cholesterol 1 mg ● Sodium 13 mg ● Carbohydrate 14.8 g ● Dietary Fiber 3.8 g ● Sugars 2.2 g ● Protein 2.4 g

Exchanges: 1 fruit, 2 fat

HELPFUL HINTS:

■ Fresh pineapple cubes can be found in the produce section of most supermarkets. Use the juice from the pineapple cubes to flavor the barbecue sauce.

■ If thin chicken cutlets are not available, use boneless, skinless chicken breasts and cut them in half horizontally to measure 1/4-inch thick.

■ Walnuts or pecans can be used instead of macadamia nuts.

SHOPPING LIST

Poultry
2 6-ounce boneless, skinless chicken breast cutlets (1/4-inch thick)

Grocery
1 small bottle low-sodium pasta sauce ❗
1 small container macadamia nuts
2 whole-wheat rolls (2 ounces each)

Produce
1 container fresh pineapple cubes
1 package washed ready-to-eat Romaine lettuce

Staples
Olive oil spray
Dijon mustard
Sugar
Reduced-fat oil and vinegar dressing ❗
Salt
Black peppercorns

❗ SHOP SMART!

Low-sodium pasta sauce (per 1/2 cup): 112 calories, 3.5 g fat, 17.7 g carbohydrate, 39 mg sodium

Reduced-fat vinaigrette or oil and vinegar dressing (per tablespoon): 11 calories, 1.0 g fat, 4 mg sodium

HONEY-SPICED MOCK CHICKEN WINGS AND CELERY WITH BLUE CHEESE DRESSING

This meal is a variation on an American favorite: spicy chicken wings with celery and blue cheese dressing. A spicy honey sauce coats meaty and flavorful boneless, skinless chicken thighs.

Honey-Spiced Mock Chicken Wings

3 tablespoons honey

2 teaspoons prepared horseradish

1/2 tablespoon distilled white vinegar

3/4 pound boneless, skinless chicken thighs

2 slices whole-wheat bread (1 ounce each)

COUNTDOWN

- Preheat broiler.
- Make chicken.
- While chicken cooks, assemble celery dish.

1. Heat broiler, and line a baking tray with foil.

2. Mix honey, horseradish, and vinegar together in a bowl.

3. Place chicken on baking sheet, and spread half the honey mixture on the chicken. Broil 5 inches from heat for 5 minutes; turn and broil 5 more minutes. A meat thermometer should read 165°F.

4. Divide chicken between two dinner plates, and spoon remaining sauce over chicken.

5. Serve chicken with bread on the side.

Preparation time: 15 minutes ● Servings: 2

Calories 372 ● Calories from Fat 67 ● Total Fat 7.5 g ● Saturated Fat 1.9 g ● Monounsaturated Fat 2.5 g ● Cholesterol 138 mg ● Sodium 293 mg ● Carbohydrate 38.1 g ● Dietary Fiber 2.1 g ● Sugars 27.8 g ● Protein 38.1 g

Exchanges: 1 starch, 1 1/2 carbohydrate, 4 lean meat

Celery with Blue Cheese Dressing

4 cups fresh celery sticks
4 tablespoons creamy yogurt blue cheese dressing **!**

1. Divide celery between two plates, and drizzle dressing over the celery. Serve with chicken.

Preparation time: 2 minutes ● Servings: 2

Calories 82 ● Calories from Fat 44 ● Total Fat 4.8 g ● Saturated Fat 0.2 g ● Monounsaturated Fat 0.1 g ● Cholesterol 10 mg ● Sodium 302 mg ● Carbohydrate 7.0 g ● Dietary Fiber 3.2 g ● Sugars 4.7 g ● Protein 2.4 g

Exchanges: 1 vegetable, 1 fat

HELPFUL HINTS:

■ Low-fat and low-sodium blue cheese dressing is available in many supermarkets.

■ A reduced-fat vinaigrette dressing can be used instead of the blue cheese dressing.

■ Boneless, skinless chicken tenderloins can be used instead of chicken thighs.

■ Fresh celery sticks can be found in the produce section of the supermarket or cut 4-inch sticks from celery stalks.

SHOPPING LIST

Poultry
3/4 pound boneless, skinless chicken thighs

Grocery
1 bottle honey
1 bottle prepared horseradish
1 loaf whole-wheat bread
1 bottle creamy yogurt blue cheese dressing **!**

Produce
1 container fresh celery sticks

Staples
Distilled white vinegar

! SHOP SMART!

Creamy yogurt blue cheese dressing (per 2 tablespoons): 50 calories, 4.5 g fat, 1.5 g saturated fat, 140 mg sodium
[*Example*: Bold House Farms]

INDIAN-SPICED CHICKEN WITH CUMIN-SCENTED RICE AND SPINACH

Tandoori chicken, with its delicate blend of spices and intriguing aroma, is one of my favorite Indian dishes. One characteristic of this dish is that it is cooked in a special tandoor oven. Another important characteristic is the ginger, garlic, coriander, and cayenne yogurt sauce that it is cooked in. For this dinner, I have captured the essence of tandoori chicken with an easy yogurt sauce. Although not made in a special oven, the meal fills my requirement for some great Indian food that can be prepared quickly.

Indian-Spiced Chicken

1 cup nonfat plain yogurt
1/4 cup loosely packed fresh mint leaves plus
   2 tablespoons, chopped
1 tablespoon peeled and chopped fresh ginger, about
   1/4-inch piece
1 teaspoon ground coriander

Pinch cayenne
2 teaspoons canola oil
3/4 pound boneless, skinless chicken tenderloins
1/4 cup fresh diced onion
1 teaspoon minced garlic

COUNTDOWN

- Place water for rice on to boil.
- Prepare ingredients.
- Start rice.
- Make chicken.
- Finish rice.

1. Mix yogurt, 1/4 cup chopped mint, ginger, coriander, and cayenne together. Heat oil in a nonstick skillet just large enough to hold chicken in one layer over medium-high heat.

2. Add chicken and onion to the skillet. Brown chicken 2 minutes; turn and brown 2 more minutes. Lower heat to medium. Add garlic to the skillet. Spoon yogurt sauce over chicken. Cover with a lid, and cook 3 minutes. A meat thermometer should read 165°F.

3. Sprinkle with remaining 2 tablespoons chopped mint, and serve.

Preparation time: 15 minutes ● Servings: 2

Calories 318 ● Calories from Fat 84 ● Total Fat 9.3 g ● Saturated Fat 1.5 g ● Monounsaturated Fat 4.3 g ● Cholesterol 111 mg ● Sodium 295 mg ● Carbohydrate 13.4 g ● Dietary Fiber 0.9 g ● Sugars 0.9 g ● Protein 43.7 g

Exchanges: 1/2 fat-free milk, 1/2 carbohydrate, 5 lean meat

Cumin-Scented Rice and Spinach

1/2 cup basmati rice
5 cups washed ready-to-eat spinach (5 ounces)
1 tablespoon canola oil
2 tablespoons raisins
1/2 teaspoon ground cumin
Salt and freshly ground black pepper

1. Bring a large saucepan filled with water to a boil over high heat. Add the rice, and let roll in the boiling water 10 minutes.

2. Add spinach, and immediately drain the rice, leaving 2 tablespoons water in the saucepan.

3. Add the oil to the saucepan, and return the rice to the pan. Add the raisins and cumin. Toss well. Add salt and pepper to taste and serve.

Preparation time: 12 minutes ● Servings: 2

Calories 275 ● Calories from Fat 68 ● Total Fat 7.5 g ● Saturated Fat 0.6 g ● Monounsaturated Fat 4.4 g ● Cholesterol 0 mg ● Sodium 64 mg ● Carbohydrate 47.1 g ● Dietary Fiber 2.7 g ● Sugars 5.7 g ● Protein 5.8 g

Exchanges: 2 1/2 starch, 1/2 fruit, 1 vegetable, 1 fat

HELPFUL HINTS:

■ Chicken tenderloin can be found in most supermarkets. If not available, use boneless, skinless chicken breasts and cut into 2-inch by 5-inch pieces.

■ All of the spices can be found in the spice section of the supermarket.

■ Basmati rice is a type of long-grain rice grown in the foothills of the Himalayas and is popular in India. It is fragrant and smells like popcorn while cooking. Long-grain white rice can be used instead.

■ Diced fresh onions can be found in the produce section of the supermarket.

■ A quick way to peel fresh ginger is to scrape the skin with the edge of a spoon.

SHOPPING LIST

Poultry
3/4 pound boneless, skinless chicken tenderloins

Dairy
1 carton plain nonfat yogurt

Grocery
1 bottle ground coriander
1 small bottle ground cumin
1 small package basmati rice
1 small bottle cayenne pepper
1 small box raisins

Produce
1 small bunch fresh mint
1 small piece fresh ginger
1 container fresh diced onion
1 bag washed ready-to-eat spinach

Staples
Canola oil
Minced garlic
Salt
Black peppercorns

CHICKEN DIAVOLO (ITALIAN CHICKEN IN SPICY TOMATO SAUCE) WITH ZUCCHINI CARROT GRATINÉE

Chicken Diavolo is a traditional Italian dinner that calls for a spicy tomato sauce. *Diavolo* is Italian for "devil," and this dish is meant to be spicy hot. The chicken breasts cook in minutes, and the heat is up to you. Zucchini and carrots make a colorful side dish.

Chicken Diavolo (Italian Chicken in Spicy Tomato Sauce)

1/2 teaspoon red pepper flakes
2 tablespoons flour
2 6-ounce chicken cutlets (1/4-inch thick)

Olive oil spray
2 cup bottled low-sodium pasta sauce 🗲
Salt and freshly ground black pepper

COUNTDOWN

■ Make chicken dish.
■ While chicken cooks, make gratinée zucchini and carrots.
■ If a microwave oven isn't available, bring a pot of water to a boil, and add the zucchini and carrots. Boil 1 minute, drain, and add Parmesan and walnuts.

1. Mix red pepper flakes and flour together. Roll the chicken cutlets in the flour mixture, pressing the mixture into the meat. Set aside.

2. Heat a medium nonstick skillet over medium-high heat. Spray with olive oil spray, and add chicken. Brown 1 minute; turn and brown 1 more minute.

3. Add pasta sauce. Bring to a simmer, cover with a lid, and simmer, gently, for 2 minutes; turn chicken over and simmer 2 more minutes. Add salt and pepper to taste and serve.

Preparation time: 10 minutes ● Servings: 2

Calories 348 ● Calories from Fat 84 ● Total Fat 9.4 g ● Saturated Fat 2.1 g ● Monounsaturated Fat 3.1 g ● Cholesterol 111 mg ● Sodium 239 mg ● Carbohydrate 24.4 g ● Dietary Fiber 3.7 g ● Sugars 11.4 g ● Protein 39.3 g

Exchanges: 1 1/2 starch, 5 lean meat

Zucchini Carrot Gratinée

2 cups grated zucchini (1/2 pound)
2 cups shredded or matchstick carrots (1/2 pound)
Salt and freshly ground black pepper
2 tablespoons grated Parmesan cheese
2 tablespoons broken walnuts

1. Grate zucchini in a food processor fitted with a grating blade or with a hand grater.
2. Place zucchini and carrots in a microwave-safe bowl. Microwave on high 3 minutes.
3. Remove and add salt and pepper to taste. Toss well.
4. Sprinkle Parmesan cheese and walnuts on top. Microwave 30 seconds. Divide between two dinner plates and serve.

Preparation time: 5 minutes ● Servings: 2

Calories 134 ● Calories from Fat 60 ● Total Fat 6.7 g ● Saturated Fat 1.4 g ● Monounsaturated Fat 1.1 g ● Cholesterol 4 mg ● Sodium 163 mg ● Carbohydrate 15.5 g ● Dietary Fiber 4.8 g ● Sugars 7.4 g ● Protein 5.4 g

Exchanges: 3 vegetable, 1 1/2 fat

HELPFUL HINTS:

■ Red pepper flakes can be found in the spice section of the supermarket.

■ Look for shredded carrots (sometimes called matchstick) in the produce section.

SHOPPING LIST

Poultry
2 6-ounce chicken breast cutlets (1/4-inch thick)

Dairy
1 small piece Parmesan cheese or container grated Parmesan cheese

Grocery
1 bottle red pepper flakes
1 bottle low-sodium pasta sauce !
1 package broken walnuts

Produce
1/2 pound zucchini
1 package shredded or matchstick carrots

Staples
Olive oil spray
Flour
Salt
Black peppercorns

! SHOP SMART!

Low-sodium pasta sauce (per 1/2 cup): 112 calories, 3.5 g fat, 17.7 g carbohydrate, 39 mg sodium

JACQUES PEPIN'S SUPREME OF CHICKEN WITH BALSAMIC VINEGAR AND ONION SAUCE WITH CORN AND PEAS

A dinner of chicken in a rich onion, mushroom, and balsamic vinegar sauce served over sautéed corn and peas takes only minutes to make. It was created by celebrity chef Jacques Pepin for his television show and book, *Fast Food My Way*. In an interview, I asked him what a French chef was doing using ketchup. He said a rich tomato sauce like ketchup has been used for centuries in France. I've adapted his recipe here.

Jacques Pepin's Supreme of Chicken with Balsamic Vinegar and Onion Sauce

3 teaspoons olive oil, divided
3/4 pound boneless, skinless chicken breast
Salt and freshly ground black pepper
1/2 cup fresh diced onion

1 cup sliced white button mushrooms
2 tablespoons balsamic vinegar
1/2 tablespoon ketchup
1/2 cup water

COUNTDOWN

■ Preheat oven to 300°F.
■ Prepare chicken and place in oven.
■ Make sauce.
■ Make corn and peas in same skillet as chicken.

1. Preheat the oven to 300°F.
2. Heat 2 teaspoons olive oil over high heat in a nonstick skillet large enough to hold the chicken breasts in one layer. When hot, add the chicken breasts, and sprinkle them with the salt and pepper to taste. Sauté, uncovered, for 3 minutes on each side.
3. Transfer the breasts to an ovenproof plate, reserving the drippings in the pan, and place the breasts in the oven. Continue cooking in the oven for 15 minutes. A meat thermometer should read 165°F.
4. Add the onion and mushrooms to the drippings in the pan, and cook for 1 minute over high heat.
5. Add the vinegar and ketchup, and continue cooking for 1 minute. Add the water, and cook until the liquid is reduced by half, about 3–4 minutes. Stir in the last teaspoon of olive oil.
6. Transfer sauce to a bowl, and use same skillet for the corn and peas. Remove chicken from oven, spoon sauce over top, and serve.

Preparation time: 25 minutes ● Servings: 2

Calories 293 ● Calories from Fat 102 ● Total Fat 11.3 g ● Saturated Fat 1.9 g ● Monounsaturated Fat 6.2 g ● Cholesterol 108 mg ● Sodium 245 mg ● Carbohydrate 8.6 g ● Dietary Fiber 1.0 g ● Sugars 4.1 g ● Protein 37.8 g

Exchanges: 2 vegetable, 5 lean meat, 1/2 fat

Corn and Peas

2 teaspoons olive oil
1 1/2 cups frozen corn kernels
1 1/2 cups frozen baby peas
Salt and freshly ground black pepper
1 tablespoon chopped fresh chives (*optional*)

1. Heat olive oil in the same skillet used for the chicken over high heat.
2. Add the corn, peas, and salt and pepper to taste. Sauté for 4 minutes, until the vegetables are cooked through.
3. Sprinkle with chives (*optional*) and serve with chicken.

Preparation time: 5 minutes ● Servings: 2

Calories 218 ● Calories from Fat 57 ● Total Fat 6.4 g ● Saturated Fat 1.1 g ● Monounsaturated Fat 3.8 g ● Cholesterol 0 mg ● Sodium 137 mg ● Carbohydrate 35.2 g ● Dietary Fiber 6.7 g ● Sugars 12.7 g ● Protein 9.2 g

Exchanges: 2 starch, 1 fat

HELPFUL HINTS:

■ Diced fresh onions can be found in the produce section of the supermarket.

■ Dried chives (1 teaspoon) can be used instead of fresh chives.

■ To save yourself from having to wash a second skillet, use same skillet to cook the chicken, corn, and peas. When the sauce is done, pour it into a bowl while the chicken bakes, and add the peas and corn to the skillet.

SHOPPING LIST

Poultry
3/4 pound boneless, skinless chicken breast

Grocery
1 bottle ketchup
1 package frozen corn kernels
1 package frozen baby peas

Produce
1 container fresh diced onion
1 container sliced white button mushrooms
1 bunch fresh chives (*optional*)

Staples
Olive oil
Balsamic vinegar
Salt
Black peppercorns

MARSALA-GLAZED CHICKEN WITH ROMAN SPINACH

The rich, smoky flavor of Sicily's Marsala wine is a key component of this quick glaze for the chicken. It brings a touch of sunny Italy to your table. Orzo is used in the Roman Spinach. It is a rice-shaped pasta.

Marsala-Glazed Chicken

3/4 pound boneless, skinless chicken breast cutlets
  (1/4-inch thick)
2 teaspoons olive oil

Salt and freshly ground black pepper
1/2 cup medium dry Marsala wine
2 tablespoons half and half

COUNTDOWN

■ Place water for orzo on to boil.
■ Prepare ingredients.
■ Boil orzo.
■ Make chicken.
■ Drain orzo and use the same saucepan for the spinach.

1. Remove visible fat from chicken. Heat oil in a nonstick skillet over medium-high heat. Brown chicken 2 minutes; turn and brown 2 more minutes. Add salt and pepper to taste.

2. Lower heat to medium, and add Marsala wine to pan. Cover with a lid, and continue to cook for 3–4 minutes. A meat thermometer should read 165°F.

3. Transfer chicken to two plates.

4. Continue to simmer sauce, about 2 minutes or until sauce is reduced by half. Add half and half. Spoon sauce over the chicken and serve.

Preparation time: 15 minutes ● Servings: 2

Calories 309 ● Calories from Fat 95 ● Total Fat 10.6 g ● Saturated Fat 2.7 g ● Monounsaturated Fat 5.1 g ● Cholesterol 114 mg ● Sodium 207 mg ● Carbohydrate 5.7 g ● Dietary Fiber 0 g ● Sugars 2.9 g ● Protein 36.6 g

Exchanges: 1/2 carbohydrate, 5 lean meat, 1/2 alcohol

Roman Spinach

1/4 cup orzo (2 ounces)
2 teaspoons olive oil
2 teaspoons minced garlic
10 cups washed ready-to-eat spinach (10 ounces)
2 tablespoons raisins
Salt and freshly ground black pepper

1. Bring a saucepan filled with water to a boil over high heat. Add the orzo, and boil 8 minutes. Drain pasta and set aside.

2. Add oil to the saucepan, and heat over medium-high heat.

3. Add garlic and spinach. Sauté 3 minutes or until spinach wilts, breaking up spinach with the edge of a spoon as it cooks.

4. Add raisins, orzo, and salt and pepper to taste. Toss well and serve.

Preparation time: 15 minutes ● Servings: 2

Calories 216 ● Calories from Fat 51 ● Total Fat 5.7 g ● Saturated Fat 0.8 g ● Monounsaturated Fat 3.4 g ● Cholesterol 0 mg ● Sodium 125 mg ● Carbohydrate 35.9 g ● Dietary Fiber 4.9 g ● Sugars 6.8 g ● Protein 8.7 g

Exchanges: 1 1/2 starch, 1/2 fruit, 1 vegetable, 1 fat

SHOPPING LIST

Poultry
3/4 pound boneless, skinless chicken breast cutlets

Dairy
1 carton half and half

Grocery
1 small bottle medium-dry Marsala wine
1 small box orzo
1 small box raisins

Produce
1 bag washed ready-to-eat spinach

Staples
Olive oil
Minced garlic
Salt
Black peppercorns

HELPFUL HINTS:

■ Buy an inexpensive Marsala wine for this recipe. It also goes well with veal, pork, and turkey. Sherry can be used as a substitute.

■ Any small pasta can be substituted for the orzo.

MEXICAN SOPE (LAYERED OPEN TORTILLA SANDWICH)

This traditional Mexican dish features little corn tortillas (*sopes*) filled with a spicy black bean spread, chicken, lettuce, and cheese. Although sopes are usually served as appetizers, they can be made into a quick and easy supper. Here's an adapted version of this Mexican favorite.

Mexican Sopes (Layered Open Tortilla Sandwich)

Olive oil spray
3/4 pound boneless, skinless chicken breasts, cut into 1/2-inch strips
Salt and freshly ground black pepper
6 6-inch corn tortillas

3/4 cup spicy black bean dip 🔒
1 cup washed ready-to-eat shredded lettuce
1/4 cup shredded reduced-fat Mexican-style cheese 🔒
1/2 cup tomato salsa 🔒

COUNTDOWN

■ Cook chicken and prepare remaining ingredients.
■ Make sope.

1. Heat a nonstick skillet over medium-high heat, and spray with olive oil spray. Add chicken, and sauté 3–4 minutes or until chicken strips are cooked. Transfer to a plate. Add salt and pepper to taste.

2. Heat the same skillet over medium-high heat, and spray with olive oil spray. Add the tortillas; warm for 30 seconds. Turn them over, and spread with the black bean dip.

3. Layer lettuce, cheese, and chicken over each tortilla. Transfer to dinner plates. Spoon salsa on top or serve on the side.

Preparation time: 10 minutes ● Servings: 2

Calories 562 ● Calories from Fat 122 ● Total Fat 13.5 g ● Saturated Fat 3.5 g ● Monounsaturated Fat 5.6 g ● Cholesterol 117 mg ● Sodium 785 mg ● Carbohydrate 57.8 g ● Dietary Fiber 11.7 g ● Sugars 4.5 g ● Protein 51.4 g

Exchanges: 3 starch, 1 vegetable, 6 lean meat, 1 fat

HELPFUL HINTS:

- Any type of salsa can be used. Choose the heat of the salsa according to your preference.
- If black bean dip is not available, use fat-free refried beans.
- Buy washed ready-to-eat shredded lettuce.
- If six tortillas don't fit into your skillet, cook them in batches or use two skillets.

PISTACHIO-CRUSTED CHICKEN AND BROCCOLI FARFALLE

These chicken breasts get a nice crunch from a chopped pistachio coating. Farfalle is a bow-tie–shaped pasta. Cooking broccoli florets with the pasta will save you a step.

Pistachio-Crusted Chicken

1/4 teaspoon salt

1/4 teaspoon freshly ground black pepper

Pinch cayenne pepper

3/4 pound boneless, skinless chicken breast cutlets, about 1/2-inch thick

3 tablespoons coarsely chopped pistachios

2 tablespoons coarse cornmeal

1 egg white, lightly beaten

Olive oil spray

COUNTDOWN

- Place a large pot of water on to boil for the pasta.
- Preheat oven to 400°F.
- Make chicken.
- Cook pasta and broccoli.

1. Preheat oven to 400°F.

2. Mix salt, black pepper, and cayenne together. Roll chicken in mixture until coated.

3. Mix pistachios and cornmeal together. Dip chicken into the egg white and then roll in pistachio mixture.

4. Heat a nonstick skillet with an ovenproof handle over medium-high heat, and spray with olive oil spray. Brown chicken breasts for 2 minutes; turn and brown 2 more minutes.

5. When chicken is golden on both sides, place skillet in oven for 5 minutes. A meat thermometer should read 165°F. Remove from oven and serve with farfalle.

Preparation time: 15 minutes ● Servings: 2

Calories 330 ● Calories from Fat 110 ● Total Fat 12.2 g ● Saturated Fat 2.0 g ● Monounsaturated Fat 5.6 g ● Cholesterol 108 mg ● Sodium 520 mg ● Carbohydrate 12.7 g ● Dietary Fiber 1.9 g ● Sugars 1.3 g ● Protein 41.6 g

Exchanges: 1 carbohydrate, 6 lean meat

Broccoli Farfalle

1/4 pound farfalle (bow tie pasta)
2 cups broccoli florets (5 ounces)
2 teaspoons olive oil
1 tablespoon lemon juice
1 teaspoon minced garlic
Salt and freshly ground black pepper

1. Bring a large pot with 3–4 quarts of water to a boil over high heat. Add pasta, and cook 5 minutes.
2. Add broccoli, and continue to cook 5 minutes. Drain, leaving about 1/4 cup water in the pot.
3. Add the olive oil, lemon juice, and garlic to the reserved cooking water.
4. Return pasta and broccoli to pot, and toss to mix well with the sauce. Add salt and pepper to taste and serve.

Preparation time: 15 minutes ● Servings: 2

Calories 277 ● Calories from Fat 51 ● Total Fat 5.7 g ● Saturated Fat 0.8 g ● Monounsaturated Fat 3.4 g ● Cholesterol 0 mg ● Sodium 23 mg ● Carbohydrate 47.9 g ● Dietary Fiber 1.9 g ● Sugars 1.7 g ● Protein 9.8 g

Exchanges: 3 starch, 1 vegetable, 1/2 fat

HELPFUL HINTS:

■ Walnuts, pecans, or macadamia nuts can be substituted for pistachios.

■ Use broccoli florets. Cut them in half if they are too large.

■ Any type of thick-cut pasta, such as elbow macaroni, can be used instead of bow ties.

SHOPPING LIST

Poultry
3/4 pound boneless, skinless chicken breast cutlets

Grocery
1 small bottle cayenne pepper
1 package shelled unsalted pistachios
1 package coarse cornmeal
1 package farfalle (bow tie pasta)
1 bottle lemon juice

Produce
1 package broccoli florets (at least 5 ounces)

Staples
Olive oil
Olive oil spray
Egg
Minced garlic
Salt
Black peppercorns

POACHED CHICKEN WITH FRESH TOMATO MAYONNAISE SAUCE AND CUCUMBER RICE SALAD

Dress up chicken with this fresh tomato-mayonnaise sauce. Poaching the chicken and letting it cool in the liquid keeps the chicken juicy and moist. It can be served hot or cold and, with this cooking method, it keeps well and tastes great the second day. Mayonnaise gets a refreshing boost from the fresh tomato pulp in this sauce. Process the tomato seeds and pulp in a food processor and cut the outer flesh into cubes for topping the chicken.

Poached Chicken with Tomato Mayonnaise Sauce

3/4 pound boneless, skinless chicken breast
1 cup fat-free, low-sodium chicken broth
  (only used for poaching liquid)
1 large tomato

1/4 cup reduced-fat mayonnaise
Salt and freshly ground black pepper
1/2 teaspoon dried tarragon

COUNTDOWN

- Start chicken.
- Make rice.
- Make sauce for chicken.

1. Place chicken in a small saucepan. Add the chicken broth. The chicken should be covered with broth. If not, add water to cover chicken.

2. Bring the broth to a gentle simmer over low heat and cook chicken 10 minutes. Do not bring the liquid to a hard boil.

3. Remove pan from the heat, and let the chicken cool down in the broth for 5 minutes. A meat thermometer should read 165°F.

4. While chicken cooks, cut the tomato in half, scoop out the seeds and pulp. Process in a food processor or blender. There should be about 1/2 cup liquid. If not add a little low-sodium tomato juice to make up the difference. Cut the tomato flesh into cubes. There should be about 1 cup cubes.

5. Mix the tomato juice with the mayonnaise until smooth. Remove chicken from broth; save 1/4 cup broth for the rice. Sprinkle chicken with salt and pepper to taste. Place on two dinner plates and spoon mayonnaise sauce over the top.

6. Sprinkle with tarragon and the tomato cubes and serve.

Preparation time: 20 minutes ● Servings: 2

Calories 315 ● Calories from Fat 131 ● Total Fat 14.6 g ● Saturated Fat 2.6 g ● Monounsaturated Fat 3.8 g ● Cholesterol 118 mg ● Sodium 435 mg ● Carbohydrate 7.9 g ● Dietary Fiber 1.7 g ● Sugars 4.9 g ● Protein 37.8 g

Exchanges: 1/2 vegetable, 4 lean meat, 2 fat

Cucumber Rice Salad

1 1/2 cups water
1 cup 10-minute brown rice (to make 1 1/2 cups cooked rice)
1 teaspoon olive oil
1/4 cup broth from poached chicken
Salt and freshly ground black pepper
1 cup cucumber cubes

1. Bring water to a boil in a saucepan over high heat. Stir in rice, return to a boil, reduce heat to medium, cover with a lid, and simmer 5 minutes.

2. Remove from heat, and let stand, covered, 5 minutes.

3. Add oil, reserved 1/4 cup chicken broth from poached chicken, and salt and pepper to taste. Fluff with a fork.

4. Add cucumber, and mix into rice.

5. Spoon rice salad onto plates with chicken.

Preparation time: 12 minutes ● Servings: 2

Calories 179 ● Calories from Fat 35 ● Total Fat 3.9 g ● Saturated Fat 0.6 g ● Monounsaturated Fat 2.1 g ● Cholesterol 0 mg ● Sodium 82 mg ● Carbohydrate 35.4 g ● Dietary Fiber 2.4 g ● Sugars 0.8 g ● Protein 3.7 g

Exchanges: 2 starch, 1 vegetable

HELPFUL HINTS:

■ When using dried tarragon, make sure the bottle is less than 6 months old.

■ The tomato juice and pulp you extract from the tomato should measure 1/2 cup. If not, add a little tomato juice to make up the difference.

■ Use a whisk to blend the tomato juice and mayonnaise to make a smooth sauce.

SHOPPING LIST

Poultry
3/4 pound boneless, skinless chicken breast

Grocery
1 bottle dried tarragon
1 box 10-minute brown rice

Produce
1 large tomato
1 cucumber

Staples
Olive oil
Fat-free, low-sodium chicken broth
Reduced-fat mayonnaise
Salt
Black peppercorns

POLLO TONNATO (CHICKEN IN TUNA SAUCE)

This is an easy scaled-down version of a traditional Italian recipe, *vitello tonnato* (veal in tuna sauce), using sautéed chicken instead of veal. It is a perfect dish to serve hot or cold. The chicken and sauce are served on a bed of red peppers and beans, making this a quick one-dish dinner.

Pollo Tonnato (Chicken in Tuna Sauce)

1/4 cup drained, water-packed white-meat tuna (about 2 ounces)

1/4 cup reduced-fat mayonnaise

1/4 cup nonfat plain yogurt

1/4 cup water

1 tablespoon olive oil, divided

2 5-ounce boneless, skinless chicken breasts

Salt and freshly ground black pepper

1 medium red bell pepper, thinly sliced (2 cups)

1 cup canned cannellini beans, drained and rinsed

1 teaspoon minced garlic

1 tablespoon capers, drained and rinsed

4 pitted black olives, cut in half

2 slices whole-grain bread (1 ounce each)

COUNTDOWN

■ Make tuna sauce.

■ Sauté chicken, peppers, and beans.

1. Place tuna in the bowl of a food processor with mayonnaise and yogurt. Process until smooth. Add water, and process to blend.

2. Heat 1 teaspoon oil in a large nonstick skillet over medium-high heat. Add chicken breasts, and brown 3 minutes; turn and brown the other side 2 minutes. Season the cooked side with salt and pepper.

3. Lower heat to medium-high, push chicken to one side, and add 2 remaining teaspoons olive oil. Add red pepper, beans, and garlic. Sauté 5 minutes, tossing beans and peppers together, stirring occasionally. A meat thermometer should read 165°F.

4. To serve, spoon the beans and peppers on individual plates, and place the chicken on top. Pour the sauce over the chicken. Sprinkle the capers and olives on top. Serve with the bread.

Preparation time: 15 minutes ● Servings: 2

Calories 557 ● Calories from Fat 133 ● Total Fat 14.7 g ● Saturated Fat 2.6 g ● Monounsaturated Fat 7.1 g ● Cholesterol 103 mg ● Sodium 611 mg ● Carbohydrate 51.9 g ● Dietary Fiber 11.9 g ● Sugars 8.4 g ● Protein 53.5 g

Exchanges: 2 1/2 starch, 1 vegetable, 6 lean meat, 1 fat

HELPFUL HINTS:

■ Great Northern or navy beans can be used instead of cannellini beans.

SHERRY CHICKEN AND GREEN BEAN PIMENTO RICE

Sherry, red peppers, and garlic are traditional Spanish ingredients. When added to chicken and rice, they make for a tasty, quick Spanish dinner. Look for skinless chicken thighs with the bone in. They have a lot of flavor, and the bone will add flavor to your sauce.

Sherry Chicken

Olive oil spray
1 pound skinless chicken thighs with bone in (yields 10 ounces meat)

2 teaspoons minced garlic
3/4 cup medium or dry sherry
Salt and freshly ground black pepper

COUNTDOWN
- Place water for rice on to boil.
- Prepare ingredients.
- Start rice.
- Make chicken.
- Finish rice.

1. Heat a nonstick skillet over medium-high heat. Spray with olive oil spray, and add chicken. Brown 2 minutes, turn, add garlic, and brown second side 2 minutes.

2. Lower heat to medium, and add sherry. Cover with a lid, and simmer 5 minutes. A meat thermometer should read 165°F. Sprinkle with salt and pepper to taste.

3. Remove chicken, and raise heat to high. Cook until sauce is reduced by half, about 2 minutes. Divid chicken between two plates and serve.

Preparation time: 15 minutes ● Servings: 2

Calories 277 ● Calories from Fat 62 ● Total Fat 6.9 g ● Saturated Fat 1.6 g ● Monounsaturated Fat 2.7 g ● Cholesterol 115 mg ● Sodium 129 mg ● Carbohydrate 9.0 g ● Dietary Fiber 0.2 g ● Sugars 0.1 g ● Protein 29.0 g

Exchanges: 1/2 carbohydrate, 4 lean meat, 1/2 alcohol

Green Bean Pimento Rice

1/2 cup long-grain white rice
2 cups trimmed green beans (1/2 pound)
1/2 cup sliced pimento, drained
2 teaspoons olive oil
Salt and freshly ground black pepper

1. Bring a large saucepan filled with 3–4 quarts water to a boil over high heat. Add rice. Boil rapidly 8 minutes.

2. Add green beans, and continue to boil 2 minutes.

3. Drain, leaving a few tablespoons of cooking water in the saucepan. Return rice to saucepan, and add pimento, olive oil, and salt and pepper to taste. Toss well and serve.

Preparation time: 15 minutes ● Servings: 2

Calories 254 ● Calories from Fat 46 ● Total Fat 5.1 g ● Saturated Fat 0.8 g ● Monounsaturated Fat 3.4 g ● Cholesterol 0 mg ● Sodium 16 mg ● Carbohydrate 47.3 g ● Dietary Fiber 5.2 g ● Sugars 2.9 g ● Protein 5.8 g

Exchanges: 2 1/2 starch, 1 vegetable, 1/2 fat

SHOPPING LIST

Poultry
1 pound skinless chicken thighs with bone in

Grocery
1 bottle medium or dry sherry
1 jar sliced pimento

Produce
1/2 pound trimmed green beans

Staples
Olive oil spray
Olive oil
Minced garlic
Long-grain white rice
Salt
Black peppercorns

HELPFUL HINTS:

■ Any type of green vegetable, such as broccoli or zucchini, can be used instead of green beans.

■ Boneless, skinless chicken breasts can be used.

■ Buy sliced pimentos or pimento strips in a jar.

■ Trimmed green beans can be found in the produce department of the supermarket.

TARRAGON CHICKEN WITH ORZO AND CHIVES

Fresh herbs, poultry, and a little vermouth are all you need for this simple, flavorful French dish. Use a skillet that just fits the chicken in one layer. If it is too large, the sauce will evaporate.

Tarragon Chicken

2 tablespoons flour
2 6-ounce boneless, skinless chicken breasts
2 teaspoons olive oil
1/2 cup sliced carrots
1/2 cup fresh sliced onion

2/3 cup dry vermouth
2/3 cup fat-free, low-sodium chicken broth
Salt and freshly ground black pepper
1 1/2 teaspoons dried tarragon
1 tablespoon half and half

COUNTDOWN

- Place a pot of water for pasta on to boil first.
- Prepare chicken.
- Finish pasta.

1. Place flour on a plate.
2. Remove visible fat from chicken, and press both sides of chicken breasts into the flour. Shake off excess flour.
3. Heat the oil in a medium nonstick skillet, just large enough to hold chicken in one layer, over medium-high heat. Add chicken, carrots, and onion. Brown chicken 3 minutes; turn and brown 3 more minutes. Transfer chicken to a plate.
4. Add vermouth to skillet. Let reduce for about 30–40 seconds.
5. Add chicken broth. Reduce by half, about 1 minute. Add salt and pepper to taste.
6. Return chicken to pan and finish cooking, about 3–4 minutes. A meat thermometer should read 165°F. Transfer to the plate.
7. Sprinkle tarragon into sauce, and cook a few seconds to warm. Add half and half, and mix well. Spoon sauce over chicken and serve.

Preparation time: 15 minutes ● Servings: 2

Calories 339 ● Calories from Fat 90 ● Total Fat 10.0 g ● Saturated Fat 2.2 g ● Monounsaturated Fat 4.9 g ● Cholesterol 111 mg ● Sodium 414 mg ● Carbohydrate 13.4 g ● Dietary Fiber 1.7 g ● Sugars 3.0 g ● Protein 39.0 g

Exchanges: 1 carbohydrate, 5 lean meat, 1/2 alcohol

Orzo and Chives

1/2 cup orzo
1 teaspoon olive oil
2 tablespoons chopped chives
Salt and freshly ground black pepper

1. Bring 3–4 quarts of water to a boil over high heat. Add orzo. Boil for 8–9 minutes after the water returns to a boil.
2. Transfer 2 tablespoons water to a bowl. Add olive oil, and mix together.
3. Drain orzo, and add to a bowl with the chives. Mix well, and add salt and pepper to taste. Serve.

Preparation time: 12 minutes ● Servings: 2

Calories 232 ● Calories from Fat 28 ● Total Fat 3.1 g ● Saturated Fat 0.5 g ● Monounsaturated Fat 1.7 g ● Cholesterol 0 mg ● Sodium 3 mg ● Carbohydrate 42.7 g ● Dietary Fiber 1.9 g ● Sugars 1.5 g ● Protein 7.5 g

Exchanges: 3 starch

HELPFUL HINTS:

■ Make sure the dried tarragon leaves are still green, not gray or brown.

■ Sliced fresh onions can be found in the produce section of the supermarket.

■ Orzo is a tiny, rice-shaped pasta. Other small pasta can be substituted.

■ A quick way to chop chives is to snip them with scissors.

SHOPPING LIST

Poultry
2 6-ounce boneless, skinless chicken breasts

Dairy
1 carton half and half

Grocery
1 small bottle dry vermouth
1 can fat-free, low-sodium chicken broth
1 bottle dried tarragon
1 box orzo

Produce
1 container fresh sliced onion
1 container sliced carrots
1 bunch chives

Staples
Flour
Olive oil
Salt
Black peppercorns

THAI CHICKEN KABOBS WITH BROWN RICE

This spicy Thai treat is easy to make. Be sure to use a good-quality Thai peanut sauce. My secret for cooking these kabobs is to leave about 1/4 inch between the ingredients on kabob skewers. This gives the heat a chance to reach all around the food. If you have short skewers, use a few more.

Thai Chicken Kabobs

3/4 pound boneless, skinless chicken breast

1 green bell pepper, seeded and cut into 8 2-inch pieces (about 1 cup)

1/2 pound yellow squash, cut into 8 slices (about 2 1/4 cups)

8 cherry tomatoes (1 cup)

Olive oil spray

2 tablespoons Thai peanut sauce

COUNTDOWN

■ Preheat boiler.
■ Prepare ingredients.
■ Start kabobs.
■ While kabobs broil, make rice.

1. Preheat broiler, and line a baking tray with foil.
2. Cut chicken into 1 1/2-inch cubes. Seed the green bell pepper and cut into 8 pieces. Wash, remove stem end, and cut yellow squash into 8 slices.
3. Thread ingredients onto two skewers, alternating between the vegetables and chicken, and place on the baking tray.
4. Spray with olive oil spray.
5. Broil 5 inches from the heat for 5 minutes. Turn and broil 3 more minutes. A meat thermometer should read 165°F.
6. Transfer to two dinner plates, and spoon 1 tablespoon peanut sauce over each kabob. Serve over rice.

Preparation time: 12 minutes ● Servings: 2

Calories 301 ● Calories from Fat 81 ● Total Fat 9.0 g ● Saturated Fat 1.7 g ● Monounsaturated Fat 3.4 g ● Cholesterol 108 mg ● Sodium 522 mg ● Carbohydrate 15.3 g ● Dietary Fiber 4.2 g ● Sugars 8.7 g ● Protein 40.6 g

Exchanges: 1/2 carbohydrate, 2 vegetable, 5 lean meat

Brown Rice

1 small package microwaveable brown rice (to make 1 1/2 cups)
1 tablespoon olive oil
Salt and freshly ground black pepper

1. Microwave rice according to package instructions.

2. Measure 1 1/2 cups cooked rice into a bowl. Reserve remaining rice for another meal.

3. Add olive oil and salt and pepper to taste. Toss well, and serve with the kabobs.

Preparation time: 5 minutes ● Servings: 2

Calories 240 ● Calories from Fat 84 ● Total Fat 9.3 g ● Saturated Fat 1.3 g ● Monounsaturated Fat 5.7 g ● Cholesterol 0 mg ● Sodium 11 mg ● Carbohydrate 29.3 g ● Dietary Fiber 1.5 g ● Sugars 0 g ● Protein 3.8 g

Exchanges: 2 starch, 1 1/2 fat

HELPFUL HINTS:

■ Zucchini can be used instead of yellow squash.

■ Remove food from skewers, and serve over the rice. Then drizzle Thai Peanut Sauce on top.

SHOPPING LIST

Poultry
3/4 pound boneless, skinless chicken breast

Grocery
1 bottle Thai peanut sauce ▯
1 package microwaveable brown rice

Produce
1 green bell pepper
1 package cherry tomatoes
1/2 pound yellow squash

Staples
Olive oil spray
Olive oil
Salt
Black peppercorns

▮ SHOP SMART!

Thai peanut sauce (per tablespoon): 30 calories, 1.3 g fat, 3.2 g carbohydrate, 311 mg sodium [*Example*: Sanjay]

TURKEY AND APPLE SALAD WITH HERBED CHEESE CROSTINI

This is a quick autumn or winter salad supper. Change the fruit to berries or peaches and serve as a cool summer supper.

Crostini is Italian for "little crusts." These are toasted rounds of bread. They're topped with herbed goat cheese in this recipe.

Turkey and Apple Salad

Olive oil spray
3/4 pound turkey tenderloin cutlets
1 1/2 tablespoons reduced-fat mayonnaise
3 tablespoons nonfat plain yogurt
3 tablespoons orange marmalade

2 teaspoons lemon juice
Salt and freshly ground black pepper
2 cups fresh apple slices
Several red lettuce leaves

COUNTDOWN

■ Preheat broiler or toaster oven.
■ Make salad.
■ Make crostini.

1. Heat a nonstick skillet over medium-high heat.
2. Spray with olive oil spray, and add turkey cutlets. Cover and cook 2 minutes; turn, cover, and cook 2 more minutes. Lower heat to medium, and cook, covered, 3 minutes.
3. While turkey cooks, mix mayonnaise, yogurt, marmalade, and lemon juice together in a medium bowl.
4. Transfer turkey to a carving board, and add salt and pepper to taste. Cut turkey into 1-inch strips. Add to a bowl, along with apple slices. Add the sauce, and toss.
5. Arrange lettuce leaves on two dinner plates. Spoon turkey salad on top and serve.

Preparation time: 10 minutes ● Servings: 2

Calories 408 ● Calories from Fat 65 ● Total Fat 7.3 g ● Saturated Fat 1.3 g ● Monounsaturated Fat 2.6 g ● Cholesterol 112 mg ● Sodium 188 mg ● Carbohydrate 42.7 g ● Dietary Fiber 3.5 g ● Sugars 13.9 g ● Protein 44.1 g

Exchanges: 1 fruit, 2 carbohydrate, 5 lean meat

Herbed Cheese Crostini

1/4 French baguette
Olive oil spray
1 tablespoon garlic-herbed goat cheese (1/2 ounce)

1. Preheat broiler or toaster oven. Cut bread on the diagonal into two slices.
2. Spray with olive oil spray. Place under broiler for 1 1/2 minutes to toast.
3. Spread with cheese and serve.

Preparation time: 5 minutes ● Servings: 2

Calories 115 ● Calories from Fat 39 ● Total Fat 4.3 g ● Saturated Fat 1.8 g
● Monounsaturated Fat 1.8 g ● Cholesterol 6 mg ● Sodium 174 mg ●
Carbohydrate 15.1 g ● Dietary Fiber 1.0 g ● Sugars 0 g ● Protein 4.0g

Exchanges: 1 starch, 1 fat

HELPFUL HINTS:

■ Boneless, skinless chicken cutlets can be used instead of turkey cutlets.

■ Fresh apple slices are available in the produce section of the supermarket.

■ Any spreadable herbed cheese can be used for the crostini.

■ Any type of bread can be used for the crostini.

■ Any type of lettuce can be used.

■ Use a toaster oven to warm the crostini.

SHOPPING LIST

Poultry
3/4 pound turkey tenderloin cutlets

Dairy
1/2 ounce garlic-herbed goat cheese
1 carton nonfat plain yogurt

Grocery
1 small French baguette
1 jar orange marmalade
1 bottle lemon juice

Produce
1 bag sliced apples
1 small head red lettuce

Staples
Olive oil spray
Reduced-fat mayonnaise
Salt
Black peppercorns

TURKEY NORMANDY WITH SWEET POTATOES

Normandy is known for its apples, cheese, and cream products—a great combination for this pan-sautéed turkey tenderloin.

Leeks need to be cleaned before cooking because sand can accumulate between the leaves. The best way to do this is to cut the leeks in half lengthwise and let water run down between the leaves.

Canned sweet potatoes finish the meal. Be sure to rinse and drain them well.

Turkey Normandy

Olive oil spray
3/4 pound turkey tenderloin
Salt and freshly ground black pepper
1 cup fresh diced onion
1 cup leek, washed and sliced (1 leek)

1 cup fresh apple slices
3/4 cup apple juice, divided
1 teaspoon cornstarch
3 tablespoons half and half

COUNTDOWN

- Prepare ingredients.
- Make turkey.
- Warm potatoes.

1. Heat a nonstick skillet over medium-high heat, and spray with olive oil spray.
2. Add turkey, and brown 2 minutes; turn and brown 2 more minutes. Sprinkle with salt and pepper to taste.
3. Lower heat to medium, and add onion, leek, and apple to skillet. Sauté, covered, for 3 minutes; turn apples over, cover, and sauté 2 minutes.
4. Mix 1 tablespoon apple juice with cornstarch until smooth, and set aside. Add remaining apple juice to the pan, scraping up any brown bits in the bottom of the skillet. Bring liquid to a simmer, cover, and cook 2 minutes. Transfer tenderloin to a carving board. A meat thermometer should read 165°F. Let it rest while you make the sauce.
5. Add cornstarch mixture to the skillet, and simmer until sauce thickens, about 1 minute. Stir in half and half.
6. Slice turkey, and spoon sauce with apples and leeks on top and serve.

Preparation time: 15 minutes ● Servings: 2

Calories 377 ● Calories from Fat 56 ● Total Fat 6.2 g ● Saturated Fat 2.4 g ● Monounsaturated Fat 2.5 g ● Cholesterol 117 mg ● Sodium 111 mg ● Carbohydrate 36.0 g ● Dietary Fiber 3.7 g ● Sugars 20.0 g ● Protein 44.3 g

Exchanges: 1 1/2 fruit, 1/2 carbohydrate, 1 vegetable, 5 lean meat

Sweet Potatoes

1/2 pound canned sweet potatoes, rinsed and drained ▯
1 tablespoon olive oil
Salt and freshly ground black pepper

1. Place potatoes in a microwave-safe bowl, and microwave on high 2 minutes to warm through.
2. Add olive oil and salt and pepper to taste and serve.

Preparation time: 3 minutes ● Servings: 2

Calories 174 ● Calories from Fat 66 ● Total Fat 7.3 g ● Saturated Fat 0.9 g ● Monounsaturated Fat 4.9 g ● Cholesterol 0 mg ● Sodium 40.7 mg ● Carbohydrate 26.8 g ● Dietary Fiber 3.2 g ● Sugars 5.9 g ● Protein 1.6 g

Exchanges: 2 starch, 1/2 fat

HELPFUL HINTS:

■ Boneless, skinless chicken can be used instead of turkey tenderloin.

■ Fresh sliced apples can be found in the produce department of the supermarket.

■ Fresh diced onions can be found in the produce section of the supermarket.

SHOPPING LIST

Poultry
3/4 pound turkey tenderloin

Dairy
1 carton half and half

Grocery
1 small bottle apple juice
1 can sweet potatoes ▯

Produce
1 container fresh diced onion
1 bag sliced apples
1 leek

Staples
Olive oil
Olive oil spray
Cornstarch
Salt
Black peppercorns

▯ **SHOP SMART!**

Canned sweet potatoes (per cup): 212 calories, 1 g fat, 50 g carbohydrate, 76 mg sodium

TURKEY PICADILLO WITH BROWN RICE

Picadillo is a popular Latin American dish consisting of ground meat, onions, green bell pepper, tomato sauce, capers, and raisins. The success of this dish arises from the blend of sweet and savory flavors. I have captured the essence of that taste and texture in this 10-minute no-fuss dinner. It takes a few minutes to gather the ingredients, but they all cook together in less than 10 minutes.

Turkey Picadillo

1 teaspoon canola oil
1 cup frozen, diced, or chopped onion
1 cup frozen, diced, or chopped green bell pepper
1 teaspoon minced garlic
2 cups low-sodium tomato sauce ⚡

2 tablespoons Worcestershire sauce
2 tablespoons capers
2 tablespoons distilled white vinegar
3/4 pound ground white-meat-only turkey breast
Salt and freshly ground black pepper

COUNTDOWN

■ Start rice.
■ Make picadillo.

1. Heat the oil in a nonstick skillet over medium-high heat. Add the onion, green pepper, garlic, and tomato sauce. Cook until the sauce starts to bubble, about 2–3 minutes.

2. Add the Worcestershire sauce, capers, vinegar, and turkey. Reduce heat to medium and cook gently, breaking up turkey with the edge of a spoon, until the meat is cooked through, about 5 minutes.

3. Add salt and pepper to taste and serve.

Preparation time: 10 minutes ● Servings: 2

Calories 378 ● Calories from Fat 37 ● Total Fat 4.1 g ● Saturated Fat 0.7 g ● Monounsaturated Fat 1.7 g ● Cholesterol 108 mg ● Sodium 539 mg ● Carbohydrate 25.0 g ● Dietary Fiber 6.7 g ● Sugars 19.8 g ● Protein 47.0 g

Exchanges: 4 vegetable, 5 lean meat

Brown Rice

1 package microwaveable brown rice (1 cup cooked rice)
1 tablespoon canola oil
Salt and freshly ground black pepper

1. Microwave rice according to package instructions. Measure 1 cup; reserve remaining rice for another meal.

2. Add oil and salt and pepper to taste. Toss well and serve.

Preparation time: 3 minutes ● Servings: 2

Calories 180 ● Calories from Fat 76 ● Total Fat 8.5 g ● Saturated Fat 0.8 g ● Monounsaturated Fat 4.8 g ● Cholesterol 0 mg ● Sodium 8 mg ● Carbohydrate 19.5 g ● Dietary Fiber 1.0 g ● Sugars 0 g ● Protein 2.5 g

Exchanges: 1 1/2 starch, 1 1/2 fat

HELPFUL HINTS:

■ Fresh diced onion and green pepper can be used instead of frozen. Look for them in the produce section of the supermarket. Cook them a minute longer.

SHOPPING LIST

Poultry
3/4 pound ground white-meat-only turkey breast

Grocery
1 bottle low-sodium tomato sauce ❗
1 small bottle Worcestershire sauce
1 small bottle distilled white vinegar
1 small bottle capers
1 package microwaveable brown rice

Produce
1 package frozen, diced, or chopped onion
1 package diced or chopped green bell pepper

Staples
Canola oil
Minced garlic
Salt
Black peppercorns

❗ SHOP SMART!

Low-sodium tomato sauce (per cup; 8 ounces): 103 calories, 0.5 g fat, 21.3 g carbohydrate, 21 mg sodium

TURKEY STROGANOFF WITH EGG NOODLES

Turkey stroganoff, an old Russian classic, can be made with turkey breast meat or leftover homemade cooked turkey. If you use cooked turkey, add about 2 cups at the end of the recipe. This will allow it to warm through in the sauce. The mixture of mushrooms, tomato paste, and mustard gives the stroganoff sauce a tangy blend of flavors and a thick texture. It tastes even better the next day! If you have time, double the recipe and save the extra for another quick dinner.

Turkey Stroganoff

3/4 pound boneless, skinless turkey fillets or slices or 2 cups leftover cooked turkey
2 teaspoons olive oil, divided
1 cup fresh diced onion
3 1/3 cups sliced button mushrooms (1/2 pound)
3/4 cup fat-free, low-sodium chicken broth

2 tablespoons tomato paste
2 tablespoons Dijon mustard
1 tablespoon sour cream
Freshly ground black pepper
2 tablespoons chopped fresh parsley (*optional*)

COUNTDOWN

■ Place water for noodles on to boil.
■ Make stroganoff.
■ Make noodles.

1. If using uncooked turkey fillets, slice turkey into 1/4-inch strips. Heat 1 teaspoon oil in a nonstick skillet over medium-high heat. Brown turkey, about 2 minutes. Transfer to a plate.

2. Add second teaspoon oil and onion to skillet. Sauté 1 minute. Add mushrooms, and continue to sauté for 2 more minutes.

3. Add broth, tomato paste, and mustard. Mix thoroughly. Simmer 2–3 minutes. Taste. You may need to add a little more mustard. There should be a delicate blend of flavors. If using cooked turkey, add it now.

4. Return the turkey to the sauce, and add sour cream and black pepper to taste. Mix thoroughly. Serve over egg noodles. Sprinkle with parsley (*optional*).

Preparation time: 10 minutes ● Servings: 2

Calories 326 ● Calories from Fat 72 ● Total Fat 8.0 g ● Saturated Fat 1.9 g ● Monounsaturated Fat 4.3 g ● Cholesterol 111 mg ● Sodium 499 mg ● Carbohydrate 16.0 g ● Dietary Fiber 3.8 g ● Sugars 5.5 g ● Protein 49.1 g

Exchanges: 3 vegetable, 6 lean meat

Egg Noodles

1/4 pound flat egg noodles (about 2 1/2 cups)
2 teaspoons olive oil
3 tablespoons water from noodles
Freshly ground black pepper

1. Bring a large pot of water to a boil. Add the noodles. Boil 10 minutes.

2. Transfer 3 tablespoons cooking liquid to a mixing bowl, and add oil to the bowl.

3. Drain noodles, and add to the bowl. Add pepper to taste. Toss well.

Preparation time: 15 minutes ● Servings: 2

Calories 197 ● Calories from Fat 50 ● Total Fat 5.5 g ● Saturated Fat 1.0 g ● Monounsaturated Fat 3.6 g ● Cholesterol 9 mg ● Sodium 114 mg ● Carbohydrate 30.0 g ● Dietary Fiber 1.0 g ● Sugars 0 g ● Protein 7.0 g

Exchanges: 2 starch, 1 fat

HELPFUL HINTS:

■ Diced fresh onions can be found in the produce section of the supermarket.

■ Any type of mushrooms can be used.

■ Use a skillet that is just big enough to hold the meat in one layer. The sauce will boil away in a larger skillet.

SHOPPING LIST

Poultry
3/4 pound boneless, skinless turkey fillets or 2 cups cooked turkey

Dairy
1 carton sour cream

Grocery
1 small can tomato paste
1 jar Dijon mustard
1 small package flat egg noodles

Produce
1 container fresh diced onion
1/2 pound sliced button mushrooms
1 bunch parsley (*optional*)

Staples
Olive oil
Fat-free, low-sodium chicken broth
Black peppercorns

PORK

Balsamic Pork Scaloppini with Garlic Sweet Potatoes and Sugar Snap Peas   158

Beer-Soused Pork with Potato and Leeks   160

Brandied Apples and Pork with Egg Noodles   162

Chimichurri Pork Chops with Quick Rice and Tomatoes   164

Chinese Pork Puffs and Quick Stir-Fried Rice   166

Chinese Pan-Roasted Pork with Stir-Fried Bok Choy and Noodles   168

Dijon Pork with Red Pepper and Tomato Penne   170

Five-Spice Pork and Rice Stir-Fry   172

Ham and Lentil Soup with Country Garlic Toast   174

Herbed Grilled Pork with Tomato-Basil Pasta   176

Pan-Fried Pork with Garlic Greens with Spicy Roast Potatoes   178

Pork Chops with Apple Relish and Sweet Potatoes   180

Pork in Port Wine with Barley and Broccoli Rabe   182

Pork Medallions with Red Berry Sauce and Mixed-Herb Angel Hair Pasta   184

Pork Pita Pocket with Greek Salad   186

Roast Pork with Chunky Strawberry Salsa and Linguine with Summer Squash   188

Salsa Pork with Fresh Linguine   190

Sara Moulton's Pork Scaloppini with Broccoli and Sweet Potatoes   192

Southwestern Honey-Glazed Pork with Salsa Potato Salad   194

Whiskey Pork with Rosemary Lentils   196

BALSAMIC PORK SCALOPPINI WITH GARLIC SWEET POTATOES AND SUGAR SNAP PEAS

Sweet and tart balsamic vinegar dresses up this pork scaloppini. Sweet potato sticks and sugar snap peas add a colorful side dish.

Using the microwave oven helps speed the cooking of the potatoes and snap peas. It also means the dish they're cooked in can be used as a serving dish and then cleaned in the dishwasher. I have also given a stovetop method.

Balsamic Pork Scaloppini

3/4 pound pork tenderloin
Olive oil spray
1 cup fresh diced onion
Salt and freshly ground black pepper

1/2 cup balsamic vinegar
2 tablespoons pine nuts
2 tablespoons chopped parsley (*optional*)

COUNTDOWN

■ Microwave potatoes and sugar snap peas and set aside.
■ Make pork dish.

1. Remove visible fat from tenderloin, and cut into 2-inch slices. Flatten the slices to about 1/4-inch thickness with a meat tenderizer or the bottom of a heavy skillet.
2. Heat a nonstick skillet over medium-high heat. Spray with olive oil spray.
3. Add pork and onions to the skillet. Sauté pork 2 minutes; turn and sauté 2 more minutes. Transfer pork and onions to a plate. Add salt and pepper to taste.
4. Raise heat to high, add vinegar. Reduce liquid by half, about 1 minute. Add pine nuts, and warm through, about 1 minute.
5. Divide pork between two dinner plates. Spoon the sauce and pine nuts on top. Sprinkle parsley on top, if using, and serve.

Preparation time: 10 minutes ● Servings: 2

Calories 338 ● Calories from Fat 86 ● Total Fat 9.6 g ● Saturated Fat 2.1 g ● Monounsaturated Fat 4.0 g ● Cholesterol 108 mg ● Sodium 113 mg ● Carbohydrate 20.2 g ● Dietary Fiber 1.9 g ● Sugars 13.0 g ● Protein 39.0 g

Exchanges: 1 vegetable, 1 carbohydrate, 5 lean meat, 1/2 fat

Garlic Sweet Potatoes and Sugar Snap Peas

1 3/4 cups sugar snap peas, trimmed (1/4 pound)
1/2 pound sweet potatoes (about 2 cups potato strips)
1 teaspoon minced garlic
2 teaspoons olive oil
Salt and freshly ground black pepper

1. Peel potatoes and cut into strips about the same size as the sugar snap peas (about 2 inches by 1/2 inch).

2. *Microwave method*
Place sugar snap peas, potatoes, and garlic in a microwave-safe bowl. Microwave on high for 5 minutes.

2. *Stove-top method*
Bring a saucepan of water to a boil, and add the potatoes. Boil 3 minutes; add sugar snap peas and garlic. Boil 2 more minutes. Drain.

3. Add olive oil and salt and pepper. Toss well and serve.

Preparation time: 10 minutes ● Servings: 2

Calories 165 ● Calories from Fat 42 ● Total Fat 4.7 g ● Saturated Fat 0.7 g ● Monounsaturated Fat 3.3 g ● Cholesterol 0 mg ● Sodium 66 mg ● Carbohydrate 28.2 g ● Dietary Fiber 5.0 g ● Sugars 7.1 g ● Protein 3.6 g

Exchanges: 1 1/2 starch, 1 vegetable, 1/2 fat

SHOPPING LIST

Meat
3/4 pound pork tenderloin

Grocery
1 bottle balsamic vinegar
1 package pine nuts

Produce
1 container fresh diced onion
1 bunch parsley (*optional*)
1/4 pound sugar snap peas
1/2 pound sweet potatoes

Staples
Olive oil spray
Olive oil
Minced garlic
Salt
Black peppercorns

HELPFUL HINTS:

■ Thin-cut boneless pork chops can be used instead of pork tenderloin.

■ Green beans or snow peas can be substituted for sugar snap peas. The cooking time and method are the same.

■ Fresh diced onions are available in the produce section of the supermarket.

■ Minced garlic can be found in the produce section or condiment section of the supermarket.

BEER-SOUSED PORK WITH POTATO AND LEEKS

Juicy pork chops, potatoes, and leeks lightly coated in a beer-mustard sauce star in this one-pot meal.

Beer-Soused Pork with Potato and Leeks

2 teaspoons canola oil
2 6-ounce boneless, top loin pork chops, fat removed
2 medium leeks, cleaned and sliced (about 2 cups)
1 pound canned potatoes, drained and sliced (about 2 3/4 cups)

2/3 cup beer
2 tablespoons cider vinegar
2 tablespoons coarse-ground mustard
Salt and freshly ground black pepper
2 scallions, sliced (1/3 cup)

COUNTDOWN

■ Prepare all ingredients.
■ Make dish.

1. Heat the oil in a nonstick skillet over medium-high heat.
2. Brown chops on both sides, about 2 minutes per side. Transfer the chops to a plate and set aside.
3. Add leeks, potatoes, beer, and vinegar to the skillet. Reduce heat to medium. Cover with a lid, and simmer 5 minutes or until potatoes are warmed.
4. Add the mustard to the skillet, and stir to blend well. Return the pork chops to the skillet; cover and simmer 5 minutes or until chops are cooked through. A meat thermometer should read 160°F. Add salt and pepper to taste. Divide between two dinner plates, sprinkle the scallions on top, and serve.

Preparation time: 20 minutes ● Servings: 2

Calories 465 ● Calories from Fat 109 ● Total Fat 12.1 g ● Saturated Fat 2.4 g ● Monounsaturated Fat 5.6 g ● Cholesterol 120 mg ● Sodium 298 mg ● Carbohydrate 44.5 g ● Dietary Fiber 7.8 g ● Sugars 1.8 g ● Protein 42.8 g

Exchanges: 2 1/2 starch, 1 vegetable, 5 lean meat, 1/2 fat

HOW TO CLEAN LEEKS

Leeks look like a giant scallion, with broad, dark green leaves that are tightly wrapped around each other. This makes it difficult to clean the dirt from the leaves. The quickest way to clean them is to trim the root end and make 4–5 slits from top to bottom. Run the leaves under cold water to reach the dirt trapped between the leaf layers.

HELPFUL HINTS:

- Any type of beer can be used.
- Dijon mustard can be used instead of coarse-grain mustard.
- 3/4 pound pork tenderloin can be used instead of boneless pork chops.
- A quick way to slice scallions is to snip them with scissors.

SHOPPING LIST

Meat
2 6-ounce boneless, top loin pork
  chops

Grocery
1 can/bottle beer
1 bottle cider vinegar
2 14.5-ounce cans sliced potatoes
1 jar coarse-ground mustard (or
  Dijon mustard)
1 large can potatoes

Produce
2 medium leeks
2 scallions

Staples
Canola oil
Salt
Black peppercorns

BRANDIED APPLES AND PORK WITH EGG NOODLES

Dress up sautéed pork chops with apples caramelized with brandy in this versatile dinner. It is suitable for an evening with friends or just a normal weeknight supper. There are many varieties of apples. Both Granny Smith and Golden Delicious apples will hold their shape when cooked. I prefer the tart Granny Smith for this recipe, but either will work well.

Brandied Apples and Pork

1/2 medium Granny Smith or other tart apple (about 1/2 cup, cut into pieces)
3/4 pound thin-cut boneless pork chops (about 1/2-inch thick)
Olive oil spray

1 teaspoon cornstarch
1/2 cup apple juice, divided
1 tablespoon honey
1/4 cup brandy
Salt and freshly ground black pepper

COUNTDOWN

■ Place water for pasta on to boil.
■ Make pork dish.
■ Boil pasta.

1. Wash and core apple; then thinly slice, and cut slices into 1-inch pieces.
2. Remove visible fat from the pork.
3. Heat a medium nonstick skillet over medium-high heat, and spray with olive oil spray. Brown chops 2 minutes; turn and brown 2 more minutes. Remove from skillet. Mix cornstarch with 2 tablespoons apple juice and set aside
4. Reduce heat, and add apple, honey, and brandy to the skillet. Let cook 30 seconds. Pour the remaining apple juice into the skillet. Cook 3 minutes. Add cornstarch mixture, and cook until sauce is thick, about half a minute.
5. Add salt and pepper to taste. Serve pork with apple slices and sauce spooned on top.

Preparation time: 10 minutes ● Servings: 2

Calories 367 ● Calories from Fat 71 ● Total Fat 7.8 g ● Saturated Fat 2.1 g ● Monounsaturated Fat 3.3 g ● Cholesterol 120 mg ● Sodium 101 mg ● Carbohydrate 21.8 g ● Dietary Fiber 0.8 g ● Sugars 18.6 g ● Protein 37.5 g

Exchanges: 1 1/2 carbohydrate, 5 lean meat, 1/2 alcohol

Egg Noodles

1/4 pound wide egg noodles
2 teaspoons olive oil
2 tablespoons freshly chopped parsley
Salt and freshly ground black pepper

1. Bring a large saucepan of water to a boil. Add the egg noodles. Boil 10 minutes or until tender but firm.
2. Transfer 2 tablespoons water from the saucepan to a large bowl. Drain pasta, and add to the bowl.
3. Add the olive oil and parsley. Add salt and pepper to taste. Toss well. Serve on individual plates with the pork chops and sauce.

Preparation time: 12 minutes ● Servings: 2

Calories 198 ● Calories from Fat 50 ● Total Fat 5.5 g ● Saturated Fat 1.0 g ● Monounsaturated Fat 3.6 g ● Cholesterol 9 mg ● Sodium 116 mg ● Carbohydrate 30.2 g ● Dietary Fiber 1.1 g ● Sugars 0 g ● Protein 7.1 g

Exchanges: 2 starch, 1 fat

SHOPPING LIST

Meat
3/4 pound thin-cut boneless pork chops (about 1/2-inch thick)

Grocery
1 small jar honey
1 small bottle brandy
1 small bottle apple juice
1/4 pound wide egg noodles

Produce
1 Granny Smith apple
1 bunch parsley

Staples
Olive oil spray
Olive oil
Cornstarch
Salt
Black peppercorns

HELPFUL HINTS:

■ The alcohol from the brandy is cooked off in this recipe. However, if you prefer, omit the brandy and add 1/2 cup more apple juice.

■ Boneless, thin-cut pork chops (1/4-inch thick) are called for. If using larger chops, increase the cooking time for the chops about 5 minutes. A meat thermometer should read 160°F. Don't overcook the pork chops.

■ The noodles will stay moist with less oil if you leave a little of the cooking water on them as they drain.

CHIMICHURRI PORK CHOPS WITH QUICK RICE AND TOMATOES

This Latin favorite features chimichurri sauce over sautéed pork. Parsley, garlic, red pepper flakes, oil, and vinegar are the basic ingredients for this piquant sauce that is used throughout South and Central America.

Chimichurri Pork Chops

3/4 pound boneless pork chops

3 tablespoons chimichurri sauce ⚡

COUNTDOWN

- Make chimichurri sauce and set aside if not using bought sauce.
- Make rice.
- Cook pork and sauce.

1. Heat a nonstick skillet over medium-high heat. Add the pork chops, and brown 2 minutes; turn and brown 2 more minutes.
2. Reduce heat to medium, cover with a lid, and cook 3 minutes. A meat thermometer should read 160°F.
3. Transfer to two dinner plates, and spread chimichurri sauce over the meat.

Preparation time: 10 minutes ● Servings: 2

Calories 351 ● Calories from Fat 185 ● Total Fat 20.6 g ● Saturated Fat 3.7 g ● Monounsaturated Fat 2.3 g ● Cholesterol 120 mg ● Sodium 145 mg ● Carbohydrate 1.5 g ● Dietary Fiber 0 g ● Sugars 0.4 g ● Protein 37.8 g

Exchanges: 5 lean meat, 3 fat

Homemade Chimichurri Sauce

2 teaspoons minced garlic
3/4 cup fresh parsley leaves
Pinch red pepper flakes

1 1/2 tablespoons olive oil
2 teaspoons apple cider vinegar
2 tablespoons water

1. Add all ingredients to a food processor, and process to form a thick sauce; it will not be smooth. (If you are making this by hand, chop parsley and garlic together and then mix in the remaining ingredients.)

Quick Rice and Tomatoes

1/2 cup long-grain white rice
1 cup low-sodium canned diced tomatoes, drained ⚠
Salt and freshly ground black pepper

1. Bring a large saucepan with 2–3 quarts of water to a boil. Add rice. Boil, uncovered, about 10 minutes. Test a grain; rice should be cooked through, but not soft.
2. Drain into a colander in the sink.
3. Return rice to the saucepan, and add the tomatoes and salt and pepper to taste. Mix well.

Preparation time: 15 minutes ● Servings: 2

Calories 189 ● Calories from Fat 4 ● Total Fat 0.5 g ● Saturated Fat 0.1 g ● Monounsaturated Fat 0.1 g ● Cholesterol 0 mg ● Sodium 14 mg ● Carbohydrate 41.8 g ● Dietary Fiber 1.8 g ● Sugars 2.9 g ● Protein 4.2 g

Exchanges: 2 1/2 starch, 1 vegetable

HELPFUL HINTS

▪ The sauce can be bought ready-made in many markets. It comes in jars or may be fresh in the deli section. I have also given a recipe for making your own, just in case it is unavailable.

SHOPPING LIST

Pork
3/4 pound boneless pork chops

Grocery
1 jar/container chimichurri sauce ⚠
1 package long grain white rice
1 small can low-sodium diced
   tomatoes

Staples
Salt
Black peppercorns

⚠ SHOP SMART!

Chimichurri sauce (per tablespoon): 90 calories, 9.5 g fat, 33 mg sodium [*Example*: Badia Chimichurri Steak Sauce]

Canned low-sodium diced tomatoes (per cup): 41 calories, 9.6 g carbohydrate, 24 mg sodium

CHINESE PORK PUFFS AND QUICK STIR-FRIED RICE

Feel like Chinese food tonight? This Chinese dinner is faster and less expensive than takeout. It'll only take you a few minutes to prepare crisp stir-fried pork served in little lettuce puffs with scallions and cucumber. Use the same wok for the rice. The pan juices from the meat will flavor the rice. Fried rice is great when it is made with leftover rice.

Chinese Pork Puffs

3/4 pound pork tenderloin
2 scallions (about 1/3 cup strips)
1/2 medium cucumber (3/4 cup strips)

8 whole lettuce leaves, removed from a head of iceberg lettuce
3 tablespoons Hoisin sauce
1 tablespoon sesame oil

COUNTDOWN

■ Prepare ingredients.
■ Microwave rice.
■ Complete pork dish.
■ Stir-fry rice.

1. Remove visible fat from pork. Cut into 1/2-inch pieces.

Prepare garnishes

2. Wash and remove root end and damaged leaves from scallions. Cut into 4-inch pieces. Slice each piece lengthwise into long slivers. Place in small bowl.

3. Peel and cut cucumber into 4-inch pieces; then cut lengthwise into thin slivers. Place in another small bowl.

4. Remove lettuce leaves in whole pieces to make lettuce cups. Wash and drain. Place in large serving bowl.

5. Spoon Hoisin sauce into small serving bowl.

6. Heat a wok or skillet over high heat. Add oil, and heat until smoking.

7. Add pork. Stir-fry 3 minutes. Remove from wok.

8. To serve, place scallions, cucumber, lettuce, Hoisin sauce, and pork on the table. Take one lettuce leaf and spoon a little sauce onto it, and then add a few scallion and cucumber slivers and some meat. Roll up, and eat like a wrap.

Preparation time: 10 minutes ● Servings: 2

Calories 325 ● Calories from Fat 105 ● Total Fat 11.7 g ● Saturated Fat 2.3 g ● Monounsaturated Fat 4.3 g ● Cholesterol 108 mg ● Sodium 488 mg ● Carbohydrate 15.9 g ● Dietary Fiber 3.3 g ● Sugars 8.7 g ● Protein 38.2 g

Exchanges: 1 carbohydrate, 5 lean meat, 1 fat

Quick Stir-Fried Rice

1 package microwave brown rice (to make 1 1/2 cups cooked)
2 teaspoons sesame oil
Salt and freshly ground black pepper

1. Microwave rice according to package instructions. Measure 1 1/2 cups rice, and reserve remaining rice for another time.
2. Add oil to same wok used for pork; heat to smoking. Add rice. Toss 3–4 minutes. Add salt and pepper to taste and serve.

Preparation time: 5 minutes ● Servings: 2

Calories 220 ● Calories from Fat 63 ● Total Fat 7.1 g ● Saturated Fat 0.7 g ● Monounsaturated Fat 3.6 g ● Cholesterol 0 mg ● Sodium 11 mg ● Carbohydrate 29.3 g ● Dietary Fiber 1.5 g ● Sugars 0 g ● Protein 3.8 g

Exchanges: 2 starch, 1 fat

HELPFUL HINTS:

■ Hoisin sauce can be found in the Chinese section of the supermarket. It's made from soy beans, vinegar, sugar, and spices.

■ To remove whole leaves from a head of lettuce, remove the core by hitting the bottom of the lettuce on a counter to loosen the core. Then twist the core out. The leaves will then come off easily.

SHOPPING LIST

Meat
3/4 pound pork tenderloin

Grocery
1 bottle sesame oil
1 bottle Hoisin sauce
1 package microwave brown rice

Produce
1 bunch scallions
1 medium cucumber
1 head iceberg lettuce

Staples
Salt
Black peppercorns

CHINESE PAN-ROASTED PORK WITH STIR-FRIED BOK CHOY AND NOODLES

This roast pork dish with a soy, garlic, and honey glaze is inspired by one of my favorite Chinese dishes, Chinese barbecue pork (*char sui*). This is a streamlined version that has similar flavor but takes only 10 minutes to make.

The steamed or fresh noodles are cooked in the microwave to save time. There is no need to boil water or dirty another pot. They're then finished with the bok choy in the same skillet used to cook the pork.

Chinese Pan-Roasted Pork

3/4 pound pork tenderloin
1/2 tablespoon reduced-sodium soy sauce
1 tablespoon honey

1 teaspoon minced garlic
1 teaspoon ground ginger
1 teaspoon toasted sesame oil

COUNTDOWN

- Microwave noodles and set aside.
- Prepare remaining ingredients.
- Make pork dish.
- Cook noodles and bok choy in same skillet used for the pork.

1. Butterfly the pork. Cut it almost in half lengthwise, and open it like a book.

2. Stir together the soy sauce, honey, garlic, and ginger in a small bowl. Set aside.

3. Heat oil in a nonstick skillet over medium-high heat. Add pork, and sauté 4 minutes; turn and sauté 4 more minutes. A meat thermometer should read 160°F. Divide into two portions, and transfer to two dinner plates.

4. Remove skillet from heat. Add soy sauce mixture, toss a few seconds, and spoon sauce over pork. Do not rinse skillet. Use it to finish noodles and bok choy dish. Serve.

Preparation time: 10 minutes ● Servings: 2

Calories 244 ● Calories from Fat 54 ● Total Fat 6.0 g ● Saturated Fat 1.5 g ● Monounsaturated Fat 2.3 g ● Cholesterol 108 mg ● Sodium 225 mg ● Carbohydrate 10.0 g ● Dietary Fiber 0.1 g ● Sugars 8.7 g ● Protein 36.1 g

Exchanges: 1/2 carbohydrate, 5 lean meat

Stir-Fried Bok Choy and Noodles

1/4 pound fresh or steamed Chinese noodles (about 2 cups)
1/2 cup water
1 teaspoon minced garlic
1 tablespoon reduced-sodium soy sauce
1/2 teaspoon ground ginger
1 tablespoon toasted sesame oil
4 cups sliced bok choy
Salt and freshly ground black pepper

1. Place noodles and water in a microwave-safe bowl. Cover and heat on high 2 minutes. Remove, stir, return to microwave, and heat on high 2 more minutes. Remove and let stand, covered, until needed.

2. Mix the garlic, soy sauce, and ginger together.

3. Heat the oil in the skillet used for the meat over high heat. Add the bok choy and noodles, and toss 1 minute.

4. Add the soy sauce mixture, and toss another minute. Add salt and pepper to taste and serve.

SHOPPING LIST

Meat
3/4 pound pork tenderloin

Grocery
1 bottle reduced-sodium soy sauce
1 bottle ground ginger
1 bottle toasted sesame oil
1 jar honey

Produce
1/4 pound fresh or steamed Chinese noodles
1 bunch bok choy

Staples
Minced garlic
Salt
Black peppercorns

Preparation time: 10 minutes ● Servings: 2

Calories 232 ● Calories from Fat 79 ● Total Fat 8.7 g ● Saturated Fat 1.4 g ● Monounsaturated Fat 2.7 g ● Cholesterol 36 mg ● Sodium 368 mg ● Carbohydrate 32.0 g ● Dietary Fiber 2.6 g ● Sugars 1.3 g ● Protein 8.0 g

Exchanges: 2 starch, 1 vegetable, 1 1/2 fat

HELPFUL HINTS:

■ Any firm green vegetable such as celery or Chinese cabbage can be used instead of bok choy.

■ Steamed or fresh Chinese noodles can be found in the produce section of the supermarket.

■ Minced garlic can be found in jars in the produce or condiment sections of the supermarket.

■ Toasted sesame oil is available in most supermarkets. Plain sesame oil can be used instead.

■ Soy sauce and garlic are used in both recipes. Measure them at one time and divide accordingly.

■ Use same skillet for pork and noodles.

DIJON PORK WITH RED PEPPER AND TOMATO PENNE

A tangy Dijon mustard sauce flavors juicy, tender pork in this French-style dinner. Bell peppers and tomatoes tossed with penne pasta complete this quick meal.

For this recipe, the pork is butterflied for faster cooking. It is easy to do, or you can ask the butcher to butterfly it for you. It is simple to do; cut almost through the pork lengthwise. Do not cut all of the way through. Open it like a book. Then cut it in half crosswise to make two portions. Pork tenderloin is very lean. The secret to keeping it moist is to sear it on each side to lock in the juices.

Dijon Pork

3/4 pound pork tenderloin
2 tablespoons Dijon mustard
2 tablespoons nonfat plain yogurt

2 tablespoons reduced-fat mayonnaise
Olive oil spray

COUNTDOWN
- Place water for penne on to boil.
- Cook pasta.
- Mix Dijon sauce ingredients.
- Make pork dish.

1. Remove visible fat from pork. Cut pork almost in half lengthwise and open like a book. Cut pork in half crosswise to make two portions.
2. Mix the mustard, yogurt, and mayonnaise together, and set aside. Heat a nonstick skillet over medium-high heat, and spray with olive oil spray. Add the pork. Sauté 4 minutes; turn and sauté 4 more minutes. A meat thermometer should read 160°F.
3. Transfer pork to a plate, and remove the skillet from the heat. Add the sauce to the skillet, and stir to dissolve brown bits in skillet. Spoon sauce over pork and serve.

Preparation time: 12 minutes ● Servings: 2

Calories 268 ● Calories from Fat 97 ● Total Fat 10.7 g ● Saturated Fat 2.2 g ● Monounsaturated Fat 4.0 g ● Cholesterol 113 mg ● Sodium 375 mg ● Carbohydrate 3.6 g ● Dietary Fiber 0.5 g ● Sugars 0.8 g ● Protein 37.3 g

Exchanges: 5 lean meat, 1 fat

Red Pepper and Tomato Penne

1/4 pound whole-wheat penne pasta (about 1 1/4 cups)
1 1/2 cups fresh diced tomatoes
1 1/2 cups fresh diced bell peppers (any color)
1 teaspoon minced garlic
2 teaspoons olive oil
Salt and freshly ground black pepper

1. Fill a large saucepan with 3 quarts water, and bring to a boil. Add the pasta. Boil 9 minutes.

2. Add tomatoes, peppers, and garlic to the saucepan. Transfer 2 tablespoons cooking water to a bowl. Drain pasta and vegetables.

3. Add olive oil to the bowl. Mix well.

4. Add pasta and vegetables to the bowl. Add salt and pepper to taste. Toss well and serve.

Preparation time: 12 minutes ● Servings: 2

Calories 289 ● Calories from Fat 52 ● Total Fat 5.8 g ● Saturated Fat 0.9 g ● Monounsaturated Fat 3.4 g ● Cholesterol 0 mg ● Sodium 16 mg ● Carbohydrate 54.2 g ● Dietary Fiber 8.3 g ● Sugars 8.4 g ● Protein 10.7g

Exchanges: 3 starch, 1 vegetable, 1/2 fat

HELPFUL HINTS:

■ Any type of pasta can be used.

■ Boneless pork chops can be substituted for pork tenderloin.

■ Cook pork until a meat thermometer reads 160°F.

■ Diced fresh tomatoes and green bell pepper can be found in the produce section of the supermarket.

■ Minced garlic can be found in jars in the produce or condiment sections of the supermarket.

FIVE-SPICE PORK AND RICE STIR-FRY

Five-spice powder serves as the base for the sauce in this meal. It adds an aromatic and exotic flavor to the dishes. It is a blend of many spices, usually star anise, cinnamon, cloves, fennel seed, and Szechwan peppercorns. It can be found in the spice section of the supermarket. You only need a little for this recipe, but I like to keep it on hand to sprinkle on cooked vegetables, over rice, or in salad dressings to create unusual flavors.

Chinese recipes need a few extra minutes to assemble the ingredients, but take only a few minutes to cook. This stir-fry dinner is ready in less than 10 minutes.

Five-Spice Pork and Rice Stir-Fry

1 package microwaveable brown rice (to make 1 1/2 cups cooked)
Salt and freshly ground black pepper
1/4 cup fat-free low-sodium chicken broth
2 tablespoons rice vinegar
1 teaspoon Chinese five-spice powder
2 teaspoons minced garlic
1 tablespoon reduced-sodium soy sauce

1 tablespoon canola oil
3/4 pound pork tenderloin, cut into 1/2-inch cubes, or stir-fry pork
1 cup fresh sliced onion
1 cup fresh diced bell peppers
1 tablespoon flour
2 tablespoons slivered almonds

COUNTDOWN

■ Make rice.
■ Assemble ingredients.
■ Complete dish.

1. Cook brown rice in the microwave according to package instructions. Measure 1 1/2 cups cooked rice. Save remaining rice for another meal. Add salt and pepper to taste, and set aside.

2. Mix chicken broth, rice vinegar, Chinese five-spice powder, garlic, and soy sauce together. Set aside.

3. Heat oil in a wok or nonstick skillet over high heat. Add pork and onion, and stir-fry 2 minutes.

4. Add bell pepper, and continue to stir-fry 1 minute. Sprinkle flour over ingredients and toss.

5. Add sauce to wok, and toss 2 minutes. Transfer to a bowl.

6. Add rice to wok, and toss 1 minute. Divide rice between two dinner plates and spoon pork and sauce over rice.

7. Sprinkle almonds on top and serve.

Preparation time: 12 minutes ● Servings: 2

Calories 597 ● Calories from Fat 190 ● Total Fat 21.1 g ● Saturated Fat 3.2 g ● Monounsaturated Fat 10.6 g ● Cholesterol 120 mg ● Sodium 456 mg ● Carbohydrate 48.4 g ● Dietary Fiber 5.9 g ● Sugars 6.2 g ● Protein 46.7 g

Exchanges: 2 1/2 starch, 1 vegetable, 6 lean meat, 2 fat

HELPFUL HINTS:

- Sliced fresh onions can be found in the produce section of the supermarket.
- Diced fresh bell peppers can be found in the produce section of the supermarket.
- Minced garlic can be found in jars in the produce or condiment sections of the supermarket.
- Boneless loin pork chops can be used instead of pork tenderloin.
- White vinegar diluted with a little water can be used instead of rice vinegar.
- Leftover brown rice can be used instead of microwaving a new package of brown rice.
- Your wok or skillet should be very hot so the meat and vegetables will be crisp, not steamed.

SHOPPING LIST

Meat
3/4 pound pork tenderloin

Grocery
1 package microwaveable brown rice
1 bottle rice vinegar
1 bottle Chinese five-spice powder
1 bottle reduced-sodium soy sauce
1 package slivered almonds

Produce
1 container fresh sliced onion
1 container fresh diced bell peppers

Staples
Canola oil
Flour
Fat-free low-sodium chicken broth
Minced garlic
Salt
Black peppercorns

HAM AND LENTIL SOUP WITH COUNTRY GARLIC TOAST

This thick and hearty soup is made with lentils, ham, and tomatoes and takes only 30 minutes to make. It's a whole meal in one bowl. Soups and casseroles are great family fare, but usually take too long to make for a mid-week meal. This quick meal fits the bill.

Ham and Lentil Soup

1 1/2 tablespoons olive oil, divided
1 cup fresh diced onion
2 teaspoons minced garlic
2 ounces sliced lean ham ▉
1 1/2 cups canned low-sodium diced tomatoes, drained ▉

2 cups water
1/2 cup dried lentils
2 teaspoons ground cumin
2 tablespoons balsamic vinegar
Salt and freshly ground black pepper

COUNTDOWN

■ Start soup.
■ While soup simmers, preheat broiler and make toast.
■ Complete soup.

1. Heat 1/2 tablespoon oil in a large saucepan over medium-high heat. Add onion, and sauté 2 minutes.
2. Add garlic and ham. Sauté 2 minutes.
3. Add the tomatoes and water. Bring to a rolling boil, and slowly add the lentils so that the water continues to boil. Boil 20 minutes.
4. Add the cumin, vinegar, and salt and pepper to taste.
5. Ladle soup into two bowls. Drizzle remaining 1 tablespoon olive oil on top and serve.

Preparation time: 30 minutes ● Servings: 2

Calories 382 ● Calories from Fat 110 ● Total Fat 12.2 g ● Saturated Fat 1.8 g ● Monounsaturated Fat 8.1 g ● Cholesterol 13 mg ● Sodium 335 mg ● Carbohydrate 49.4 g ● Dietary Fiber 18.2 g ● Sugars 11.1 g ● Protein 20.9 g

Exchanges: 2 starch, 2 vegetable, 2 lean meat, 2 fat

Country Garlic Toast

1 tablespoon olive oil
2 slices crusty country bread (1 ounce each)
1 garlic clove, cut in half

1. Spread the oil over the bread, and rub cut edge of garlic on top.
2. Place under a broiler or in a toaster oven for several minutes or until bread is golden. Remove and serve with soup.

Preparation time: 5 minutes ● Servings: 2

Calories 131 ● Calories from Fat 71 ● Total Fat 7.9 g ● Saturated Fat 1.2 g ● Monounsaturated Fat 5.1 g ● Cholesterol 0 mg ● Sodium 110 mg ● Carbohydrate 11.8 g ● Dietary Fiber 2.0 g ● Sugars 1.7 g ● Protein 3.6 g

Exchanges: 1 starch, 1 1/2 fat

HELPFUL HINTS:

■ Canned whole tomatoes can be used instead of diced.

■ Diced fresh onions can be found in the produce section of the supermarket.

■ Minced garlic can be found in jars in the produce or condiment sections of the supermarket.

■ Toast can be made in a toaster oven or under the broiler.

SHOPPING LIST

Deli
2 ounces lean ham ⚠

Grocery
1 can low-sodium diced tomatoes ⚠
1 package dried lentils
1 bottle ground cumin
1 loaf crusty country bread

Produce
1 container fresh diced onion

Staples
Olive oil
Minced garlic
Garlic
Balsamic vinegar
Salt
Black peppercorns

⚠ **SHOP SMART!**

Lean ham (per ounce): 30 calories, 0.7 g fat, 0.2 g saturated fat, 301 mg sodium

Canned low-sodium diced tomatoes (per cup): 41 calories, 9.6 g carbohydrate, 24 mg sodium

HERBED GRILLED PORK WITH TOMATO-BASIL PASTA

This uncooked tomato-basil sauce is easy to make. Use a good-quality can or carton of low-sodium whole tomatoes. The sauce can also be used over any type of grilled meat or tossed with cooked vegetables. It will keep several days in the refrigerator.

The Herbed Grilled Pork can be served hot or at room temperature. I make it on a stove-top grill for a quick dinner.

Herbed Grilled Pork

3/4 pound pork tenderloin
Olive oil spray
1 teaspoon dried oregano

1 teaspoon dried rosemary
Salt and freshly ground black pepper

COUNTDOWN

- Place water for pasta on to boil.
- Grill pork.
- While pork cooks, make sauce for pasta.

1. Remove visible fat from pork. Butterfly the pork: Cut the pork almost in half lengthwise. Do not cut all the way through. Open it like a book.
2. Spray pork with olive oil spray.
3. Sprinkle oregano and rosemary on both sides.
4. Heat a stove-top grill, and grill pork for 10 minutes; turn and grill 5 more minutes. A meat thermometer should read 160°F. Remove from grill, sprinkle with salt and pepper to taste, cover with foil, and let stand for 5 minutes. Cut into slices. Serve with the pasta.

Preparation time: 25 minutes ● Servings: 2

Calories 207 ● Calories from Fat 49 ● Total Fat 5.4 g ● Saturated Fat 1.7 g ● Monounsaturated Fat 2.4 g ● Cholesterol 108 mg ● Sodium 93 mg ● Carbohydrate 1.8 g ● Dietary Fiber 0.9 g ● Sugars 0 g ● Protein 35.8 g

Exchanges: 5 lean meat

Tomato-Basil Pasta

1 1/2 cups canned plum tomatoes, drained
2 teaspoons minced garlic
2 teaspoons olive oil
2 tablespoons tomato paste
1/2 cup fresh basil leaves
1/8 teaspoon cayenne pepper
Salt
1/4 pound linguine
2 tablespoons grated Parmesan cheese

1. Place water for pasta on to boil over high heat.
2. Place tomatoes in the bowl of a food processor with the garlic, oil, tomato paste, and basil. Process until mixture has the consistency of a sauce or it is smooth. Add the cayenne and salt to taste.
3. Add pasta to boiling water. After water comes back to a boil, continue to cook 10 minutes for dried pasta or 3 minutes for fresh. Drain and place in a serving bowl.
4. Pour tomato sauce over the top, and mix thoroughly. The heat of the pasta will cook the sauce. Sprinkle the Parmesan on top and serve.

Preparation time: 15 minutes ● Servings: 2

Calories 320 ● Calories from Fat 65 ● Total Fat 7.3 g ● Saturated Fat 1.7 g ● Monounsaturated Fat 3.9 g ● Cholesterol 4 mg ● Sodium 104 mg ● Carbohydrate 53.3 g ● Dietary Fiber 4.5 g ● Sugars 7.1 g ● Protein 11.8 g

Exchanges: 3 starch, 2 vegetable, 1 fat

HELPFUL HINTS:

■ Boneless pork chops can be used instead of tenderloin.

■ The pork can be cooked under a broiler. The timing will be about the same. A meat thermometer should read 160°F.

SHOPPING LIST

Pork
3/4 pound pork tenderloin

Dairy
1 small piece Parmesan cheese

Grocery
1 bottle dried oregano
1 bottle dried rosemary
1 small bottle cayenne pepper
1 large can plum tomatoes
1 small can tomato paste
1/4 pound linguine

Produce
1 bunch basil

Staples
Olive oil
Olive oil spray
Minced garlic
Salt
Black peppercorns

PAN-FRIED PORK WITH GARLIC GREENS WITH SPICY ROAST POTATOES

Baby arugula tossed with garlic and dressing is the quick topping for these pan-fried pork chops. By cooking the pork chops in a skillet over high heat for just a few minutes, the juices are sealed in and the meat stays juicy and tender. To speed the cooking time for the pork, I buy boneless thin-cut loin chops. They are about 1/2-inch thick and can be found in most supermarkets. But any boneless pork chops can be used. Cut them almost in half horizontally, and open them like a book. Then flatten them to about 1/2-inch thick. Either works well with this recipe.

This entrée is accompanied by spicy roast potatoes. These potatoes are "roasted" under a hot broiler. Be sure to preheat the broiler before adding the potatoes. They take about 15 minutes to cook.

Pan-Fried Pork with Garlic Greens

3/4 pound boneless pork chops,
   flattened to 1/2-inch thick
Olive oil spray
1 teaspoon minced garlic

Salt and freshly ground black pepper
2 1/2 cups washed ready-to-eat baby arugula
   (2 ounces)
2 tablespoons reduced-fat vinaigrette dressing

COUNTDOWN

- Preheat broiler for potatoes.
- Prepare and roast potatoes.
- While potatoes roast, make pork recipe.

1. Remove visible fat from pork. Heat a nonstick skillet over medium-high heat, and spray with olive oil spray.
2. When skillet is very hot, add pork. Cook 2 minutes, turn, add garlic, and cook 2 more minutes. A meat thermometer should read 160°F.
3. Transfer to individual plates. Sprinkle with salt and pepper to taste.
4. Remove skillet from heat, and add arugula and vinaigrette dressing. Toss well. The leaves should be warm but still firm. Spoon over the pork. Season with salt and pepper to taste and serve.

Preparation time: 10 minutes ● Servings: 2

Calories 251 ● Calories from Fat 80 ● Total Fat 8.9 g ● Saturated Fat 2.2 g ● Monounsaturated Fat 3.6 g ● Cholesterol 121 mg ● Sodium 109 mg ● Carbohydrate 3.0 g ● Dietary Fiber 0.5 g ● Sugars 1.2 g ● Protein 38.3 g

Exchanges: 5 lean meat, 1/2 fat

Spicy Roast Potatoes

Olive oil spray
1 pound red potatoes
1/8 teaspoon cayenne pepper
Salt and freshly ground black pepper

1. Preheat broiler. Line a baking sheet with foil, and spray with olive oil spray.
2. Wash potatoes, do not peel, and cut into 1-inch pieces. Spread on baking sheet. Spray potatoes with olive oil spray. Sprinkle baking sheet with cayenne pepper.
3. Add potatoes to the sheet, and roll around to coat with olive oil spray and cayenne pepper. Sprinkle with salt and black pepper to taste.
4. Broil 5 inches from heat for 10 minutes. Remove from broiler, and turn potatoes over. Return to broiler for 5 more minutes. Remove and serve with pork.

Preparation time: 15 minutes ● Servings: 2

Calories 173 ● Calories from Fat 16 ● Total Fat 1.7 g ● Saturated Fat 0.3 g ● Monounsaturated Fat 1.0 g ● Cholesterol 0 mg ● Sodium 16 mg ● Carbohydrate 36.6 g ● Dietary Fiber 3.9 g ● Sugars 2.3 g ● Protein 4.3 g

Exchanges: 2 1/2 starch

SHOPPING LIST

Meat
3/4 pound boneless pork chops

Grocery
1 bottle cayenne pepper

Produce
2 ounces washed ready-to-eat baby arugula
1 pound red potatoes

Staples
Olive oil spray
Minced garlic
Reduced-fat vinaigrette dressing **!**
Salt
Black peppercorns

! SHOP SMART!

Reduced-fat vinaigrette or oil and vinegar dressing (per tablespoon): 11 calories, 1.0 g fat, 4 mg sodium

HELPFUL HINTS:

■ Any type of potato can be used.

■ Washed ready-to-eat arugula can be found in the produce department. Any type of firm lettuce can be used instead of arugula.

■ Minced garlic can be found in jars in the produce or condiment sections of the supermarket.

PORK CHOPS WITH APPLE RELISH AND SWEET POTATOES

Sweet and tart apple relish garnishes the sautéed boneless pork chop in this quick recipe. Sweet potatoes, gently steamed, complete this fall harvest meal.

Apples should be kept in the refrigerator and, if washed, dried thoroughly before being placed in the refrigerator. This recipe calls for a Gala apple. It's a sweet, moderately crisp, juicy apple that holds its shape well and adds just the right amount of sweetness to the relish. If you can't find Gala apples, use another type of your choice.

Pork Chops with Apple Relish

1 medium Gala apple, cored and coarsely chopped
(about 1 1/2 cups)
2 tablespoons fresh diced red onion
2 tablespoons apple cider vinegar
1 tablespoon honey

1 teaspoon canola oil
2 6-ounce thin-cut boneless loin pork chops
(1/4-inch thick)
Salt and freshly ground black pepper

COUNTDOWN

■ Start potatoes.
■ Make relish.
■ Cook pork chops.
■ Finish potatoes.

1. Mix apple, onion, apple cider vinegar, and honey together in a small bowl. Set aside.

2. Heat oil in a small nonstick skillet over medium-high heat. Add pork chops, and brown 2 minutes; turn and brown 2 more minutes. Add salt and pepper to taste. A meat thermometer should read 160°F.

3. Place pork chops on individual dinner plates. Spoon apple relish on top and serve.

Preparation time: 10 minutes ● Servings: 2

Calories 322 ● Calories from Fat 78 ● Total Fat 8.7 g ● Saturated Fat 2.1 g ● Monounsaturated Fat 3.7 g ● Cholesterol 120 mg ● Sodium 98 mg ● Carbohydrate 22.2 g ● Dietary Fiber 2.4 g ● Sugars 18.5 g ● Protein 37.8 g

Exchanges: 1 1/2 fruit, 5 lean meat

Sweet Potatoes

3/4 pound sweet potatoes, peeled and cut into 1-inch pieces
2 teaspoons canola oil
Salt and freshly ground black pepper

1. Place potatoes in a steaming basket, and place the basket over water in a saucepan. The water should not touch the bottom of the basket. Cover and steam potatoes 10 minutes.
2. Transfer potatoes to a bowl, and add canola oil. Toss, making sure all of the pieces are coated with oil. Add salt and pepper to taste. Serve with the pork chops.

Preparation time: 12 minutes ● Servings: 2

Calories 186 ● Calories from Fat 41 ● Total Fat 4.6 g ● Saturated Fat 0.4 g ● Monounsaturated Fat 2.8 g ● Cholesterol 0 mg ● Sodium 94 mg ● Carbohydrate 34.3 g ● Dietary Fiber 5.1 g ● Sugars 7.1 g ● Protein 2.7 g

Exchanges: 2 starch, 1/2 fat

HELPFUL HINTS:

■ Diced fresh onions can be found in the produce section of the supermarket.

■ Thin-cut pork chops (1/4-inch thick) are called for. If using larger chops, increase the cooking time for the chops by about 5 minutes. A meat thermometer should read 160°F.

■ Coarsely chop apples in the food processor, using the pulse button.

SHOPPING LIST

Meat
2 6-ounce thin-cut boneless loin pork chops (1/4-inch thick)

Grocery
1 bottle apple cider vinegar
1 jar honey

Produce
1 medium Gala apple
1 container fresh diced red onion
3/4 pound sweet potatoes

Staples
Canola oil
Salt
Black peppercorns

PORK IN PORT WINE WITH BARLEY AND BROCCOLI RABE

Whether you want to serve up a special weekend meal or a quick weeknight dinner, this juicy pork tenderloin, cut into medallions and sautéed in a rich port wine sauce, will not let you down. Ketchup is the secret ingredient. Thick tomato sauce has been used in French cooking for many years. It gives just the right amount of sweet and savory flavor and texture to the port-based sauce.

Pork in Port Wine

1/2 cup fat-free low-sodium chicken broth
2 tablespoons ketchup
3/4 pound pork tenderloin
1 teaspoon olive oil

Salt and freshly ground black pepper
1/2 cup port wine
1 teaspoon dried thyme

COUNTDOWN

- Prepare ingredients.
- Start the barley and broccoli rabe.
- Make pork dish.

1. Mix chicken broth and ketchup together, and set aside.
2. Remove visible fat from pork. Cut into 1-inch slices.
3. Heat olive oil in a nonstick skillet over medium-high heat. Add pork and brown 3 minutes; turn and brown 3 more minutes. Add salt and pepper to taste to cooked sides. Lower heat to medium, and cook 5 minutes. A meat thermometer should read 160°F. Transfer to two dinner plates.
4. Add the port to the skillet and bring to a boil, scraping up the brown bits as it boils for about 30 seconds.
5. Add the chicken broth and ketchup mixture, and cook about 2 minutes. Sprinkle with thyme. Spoon sauce over pork and serve.

Preparation time: 10 minutes ● Servings: 2

Calories 293 ● Calories from Fat 55 ● Total Fat 6.1 g ● Saturated Fat 1.5 g ● Monounsaturated Fat 3.0 g ● Cholesterol 108 mg ● Sodium 392 mg ● Carbohydrate 8.5 g ● Dietary Fiber 0.3 g ● Sugars 0.0 g ● Protein 36.9 g

Exchanges: 1/2 carbohydrate, 5 lean meat, 1/2 alcohol

Barley and Broccoli Rabe

5 1/2 cups broccoli rabe, stems trimmed (1/2 pound)
1 1/2 cups water
1/2 cup quick-cooking barley
2 teaspoons olive oil
Salt and freshly ground black pepper

1. Cut off thick broccoli rabe stems and discard. Cut broccoli rabe into 1-inch pieces.
2. Bring water to a boil in a medium saucepan over high heat. Add broccoli and barley.
3. Bring back to a boil, lower heat to medium-high, cover, and cook 10 minutes. Water will be absorbed.
4. Add olive oil and salt and pepper to taste and serve.

Preparation time: 15 minutes ● Servings: 2

Calories 241 ● Calories from Fat 51 ● Total Fat 5.6 g ● Saturated Fat 0.8 g ● Monounsaturated Fat 3.4 g ● Cholesterol 0 mg ● Sodium 41 mg ● Carbohydrate 42.1 g ● Dietary Fiber 10.9 g ● Sugars 0.8 g ● Protein 8.5 g

Exchanges: 2 starch, 1 vegetable, 1 fat

HELPFUL HINTS:

■ Sherry can be used instead of port.

■ Look for washed ready-to-eat arugula (also called roquette or rocket) in the produce section.

SHOPPING LIST

Meat
3/4 pound pork tenderloin

Grocery
1 small bottle port wine
1 bottle dried thyme
1 package quick-cooking barley

Produce
1/2 pound broccoli rabe

Staples
Olive oil
Fat-free low-sodium chicken broth
Ketchup
Salt
Black peppercorns

PORK MEDALLIONS WITH RED BERRY SAUCE AND MIXED-HERB ANGEL HAIR PASTA

This tangy Red Berry Sauce is simple and goes great with pork medallions. The sauce is thickened by puréeing cranberries in a blender or food processor. You'll need only a few cranberries for this recipe; you can freeze the rest for another use.

Delicate, fresh angel hair pasta takes only a minute to cook. If it cooks too long, it will clump together and taste pasty. The secret to cooking angel hair pasta is to bring the water to a rolling boil in a large pasta pot and then add the pasta. Lots of fresh herbs give this dish a fresh, garden flavor.

Pork Medallions with Red Berry Sauce

3/4 pound pork tenderloin
1 teaspoon olive oil
Salt and freshly ground black pepper
1/4 cup cider vinegar

1/2 cup cranberry juice
1 tablespoon honey
1/2 cup fresh cranberries

COUNTDOWN

■ Place water for pasta on to boil.
■ Make pork recipe.
■ Make pasta recipe.

1. Remove visible fat from pork. Cut pork into 1-inch slices to form round medallions.
2. Heat oil in a nonstick skillet over medium-high heat until smoking. Brown pork medallions for 2 minutes; turn and brown for 2 more minutes. Sprinkle salt and pepper to taste on cooked sides. Remove from pan.
3. Lower heat to medium, and add vinegar. Let simmer about 30 seconds, scraping up all of the brown bits in the pan while the liquid reduces. Add cranberry juice and honey. Stir to thoroughly combine.
4. Add cranberries, and return pork to pan. Gently simmer for 2 minutes. Turn pork and simmer another 2 minutes.
5. Transfer pork to individual plates. Pour sauce into a blender or food processor, and blend until smooth. This takes a few seconds. Spoon the sauce over the pork and serve.

Preparation time: 15 minutes ● Servings: 2

Calories 295 ● Calories from Fat 55 ● Total Fat 6.1 g ● Saturated Fat 1.5 g ● Monounsaturated Fat 3.0 g ● Cholesterol 108 mg ● Sodium 95 mg ● Carbohydrate 21.4 g ● Dietary Fiber 1.0 g ● Sugars 9.3 g ● Protein 35.8 g

Exchanges: 1 1/2 fruit, 5 lean meat

Mixed-Herb Angel Hair Pasta

3 ounces fresh angel hair pasta (1 rounded cup cooked)
2 teaspoons olive oil
2 teaspoons cider vinegar
1 cup chopped fresh basil
1/2 cup snipped fresh chives
Salt and freshly ground black pepper

1. Fill a large saucepan with water, and bring water to a boil. Add pasta. Stir and boil 1 minute. (If using dried pasta, boil 3–4 minutes.) Drain.
2. Place in a bowl or back in the saucepan, and add oil and vinegar. Toss well. Add basil, chives, and salt and pepper to taste. Toss again and serve.

Preparation time: 5 minutes ● Servings: 2

Calories 206 ● Calories from Fat 48 ● Total Fat 5.3 g ● Saturated Fat 0.8 g ● Monounsaturated Fat 3.4 g ● Cholesterol 0 mg ● Sodium 3 mg ● Carbohydrate 32.8 g ● Dietary Fiber 2.0 g ● Sugars 1.4 g ● Protein 6.4 g

Exchanges: 2 starch, 1 fat

HELPFUL HINTS:

■ Dried angel hair pasta can be used instead of fresh. Boil it for 3 minutes.

■ A quick way to chop herbs is to snip them with scissors.

■ Be sure to heat your skillet to smoking before adding the meat. The pork will brown instead of steam when it is placed in the pan.

SHOPPING LIST

Meat
3/4 pound pork tenderloin

Grocery
1 bottle cider vinegar
1 bottle cranberry juice
1 package fresh angel hair pasta

Produce
1 package fresh cranberries
1 bunch basil
1 bunch chives

Staples
Olive oil
Honey
Salt
Black peppercorns

PORK PITA POCKET WITH GREEK SALAD

Sautéed pork is garnished with a refreshing cucumber sauce and stuffed in pita bread in this quick meal. For the Greek Salad, take washed ready-to-eat salad and spice it up with cherry tomatoes, radishes, and feta cheese.

Pork Pita Pocket

3/4 pound boneless pork tenderloin, precut for stir-fry (about 2-inch by 1/2-inch strips)

3 tablespoons reduced-fat oil and vinegar dressing 🔟

1 cup fresh diced cucumber

3/4 cup nonfat plain yogurt

2 tablespoons fresh diced onion

1/2 tablespoon dried dill

2 6-inch whole-wheat pita breads

COUNTDOWN

■ Marinate pork.
■ Prepare cucumber sauce.
■ Prepare tomato and corn salsa and set aside to marinate a few minutes.
■ Make the Greek Salad.
■ Cook pork and make pita pockets.

1. Place pork in a self-sealing plastic bag. Add oil and vinegar dressing. Set aside and let stand while the other ingredients are prepared (about 5 minutes).

2. Mix cucumber, yogurt, onion, and dill together in a bowl. Set aside.

3. Heat a nonstick skillet over medium-high heat. Drain pork, reserve the marinade, and add pork to skillet. Sauté 2 minutes. Add marinade, and sauté 3 minutes. Marinade should come to a boil.

4. Cut pita breads in half, and open pockets. Fill with pork, top with cucumber dressing, and serve.

Preparation time: 15 minutes ● Servings: 2

Calories 435 ● Calories from Fat 64 ● Total Fat 7.1 g ● Saturated Fat 1.7 g ● Monounsaturated Fat 2.1 g ● Cholesterol 111mg ● Sodium 508 mg ● Carbohydrate 45.5 g ● Dietary Fiber 5.3 g ● Sugars 2.3 g ● Protein 47.8 g

Exchanges: 2 starch, 1/2 fat-free milk, 1 vegetable, 5 lean meat

Greek Salad

5 cups washed ready-to-eat salad
8 cherry tomatoes
1/2 cup radishes, trimmed and cut into quarters
2 tablespoons reduced-fat oil and vinegar dressing **!**
1 tablespoon crumbled feta cheese

1. Place salad in a bowl. Add tomatoes and radishes.

2. Add dressing and toss.

3. Sprinkle feta cheese on top and serve.

Preparation time: 5 minutes ● Servings: 2

Calories 64 ● Calories from Fat 23 ● Total Fat 2.5 g ● Saturated Fat 0.9 g
● Monounsaturated Fat 0.6 g ● Cholesterol 5 mg ● Sodium 82 mg ●
Carbohydrate 9.3 g ● Dietary Fiber 4.1 g ● Sugars 5.0 g ● Protein 3.2 g

Exchanges: 2 vegetable, 1/2 fat

HELPFUL HINTS:

■ If pork strips aren't available, use pork tenderloin and slice it into 1/4- to 1/2-inch slices and then into 5-inch long strips.

■ Fresh diced cucumber is available in the produce section of the supermarket.

■ Fresh diced onions are available in the produce section of the supermarket.

■ If you have time, use fresh dill. Snip the leaves with scissors.

ROAST PORK WITH CHUNKY STRAWBERRY SALSA AND LINGUINE WITH SUMMER SQUASH

This sweet and spicy combination features pork tenderloin with chunky strawberry salsa. Strawberries make a delicious dessert, but I also add them to salads or use them to make tasty condiments for cooked meats. Any type of berry can be used.

Strawberries are best stored in the refrigerator unwashed, in a large container lined with paper towels. Remove from the refrigerator, bring to room temperature, and wash them just before using. You can also freeze them for up to a year in an airtight bag.

Roast Pork with Chunky Strawberry Salsa

3/4 pound pork tenderloin
Olive oil spray
1 1/2 teaspoons ground cumin, divided
1 cup ripe strawberries, hulled and coarsely chopped
1 teaspoon sugar

2 tablespoons fresh diced red onion
Several drops hot pepper sauce
1 tablespoon freshly squeezed lime juice
2 tablespoons chopped fresh cilantro (*optional*)
Salt

COUNTDOWN

- Preheat broiler and baking sheet.
- Place water for pasta on to boil.
- Broil pork.
- Make salsa.
- Cook pasta and squash.

1. Preheat broiler, line a baking sheet with foil, and place under broiler.
2. Remove visible fat from pork, and spray all sides with olive oil spray.
3. Sprinkle pork with 1 teaspoon ground cumin.
4. Remove baking sheet from broiler, and place tenderloin on sheet. Broil 10 minutes; turn and cook another 10 minutes. A meat thermometer should read 160°F.
5. While pork broils, place strawberries in a medium bowl and sprinkle with sugar. Add onion and hot pepper sauce.
6. Mix the remaining 1/2 teaspoon cumin and lime juice together, and drizzle over ingredients. Add salt to taste. Toss well. Sprinkle with cilantro (*optional*) and serve pork with salsa spooned over top.

Preparation time: 15 minutes ● Servings: 2

Calories 243 ● Calories from Fat 52 ● Total Fat 5.8 g ● Saturated Fat 1.4 g ● Monounsaturated Fat 2.6 g ● Cholesterol 108 mg ● Sodium 105 mg ● Carbohydrate 10.1 g ● Dietary Fiber 2.1 g ● Sugars 2.6 g ● Protein 36.6 g

Exchanges: 1/2 fruit, 5 lean meat

Linguine with Summer Squash

1/4 pound spinach linguine
2 1/4 cups frozen sliced yellow squash (1/2 pound)
1 tablespoon olive oil
Salt and freshly ground black pepper

1. Place a large saucepan filled with 3–4 quarts of water on to boil over high heat. Add the pasta, and boil 2 minutes.

2. Add the squash. Continue to boil 8 minutes or until the pasta is cooked through but firm.

3. Drain the pasta and vegetables. Place in a bowl, and toss with olive oil. Add salt and pepper to taste and serve.

Preparation time: 15 minutes ● Servings: 2

Calories 291 ● Calories from Fat 70 ● Total Fat 7.8 g ● Saturated Fat 1.2 g ● Monounsaturated Fat 5.0 g ● Cholesterol 0 mg ● Sodium 5 mg ● Carbohydrate 46.8 g ● Dietary Fiber 3.1 g ● Sugars 4.3 g ● Protein 9.0 g

Exchanges: 3 starch, 1 vegetable, 1 fat

HELPFUL HINTS:

■ Diced fresh onions can be found in the produce section of the supermarket.

■ If you like your salsa hot, add more hot pepper sauce.

■ Placing the pork on a preheated baking sheet helps it to cook faster.

■ Coarsely chop strawberries in food processor using the pulse button.

SALSA PORK WITH FRESH LINGUINE

Spicy tomato salsa perks up pork chops in this simple recipe. This is a one-pot meal that takes only 15 minutes to cook. If you keep these ingredients on hand, you can prepare a quick dinner without having to go to the market. Keep pork and peas in the freezer, fresh pasta in the fridge, and salsa on the shelf.

Salsa Pork with Fresh Linguine

3 cups water
1/4 pound fresh linguine
1 cup frozen peas
3 teaspoons olive oil, divided
Salt and freshly ground black pepper

3/4 pound thin-cut boneless pork chops
  (1/4-inch thick)
3/4 cup chunky salsa
1/2 cup chopped parsley (*optional*)

COUNTDOWN

- Place water on to boil for the pasta.
- Prepare ingredients.
- Cook linguine and peas.
- Make pork dish.

1. Bring water to a boil in a large skillet over high heat. Add pasta and peas. Bring back to a boil for 3 minutes. Drain and transfer to a bowl. Toss with 1 teaspoon oil and salt and pepper to taste.

2. Heat remaining 2 teaspoons oil in the same skillet over medium-high heat. Add pork, and brown 2 minutes; turn and brown 2 more minutes. Sprinkle cooked side with salt and pepper to taste. A meat thermometer should read 160°F.

3. Divide linguine between two plates. Place pork on the plates, and spoon salsa on top. Sprinkle parsley over pork, if desired, and serve.

Preparation time: 10 minutes ● Servings: 2

Calories 578 ● Calories from Fat 130 ● Total Fat 14.5 g ● Saturated Fat 3.1 g ● Monounsaturated Fat 7.4 g ● Cholesterol 120 mg ● Sodium 383 mg ● Carbohydrate 59.5 g ● Dietary Fiber 6.8 g ● Sugars 8.5 g ● Protein 50.5 g

Exchanges: 3 1/2 starch, 1 vegetable, 5 lean meat, 1 fat

HELPFUL HINTS:

■ Any type of green vegetable can be substituted for the peas.

■ Dried linguine can be used. Cook the pasta for 5 minutes, add peas, and cook 4 more minutes.

SARA MOULTON'S PORK SCALOPPINI WITH BROCCOLI AND SWEET POTATOES

I asked TV chef Sara Moulton what she serves her family for a quick meal, and this is what she gave me. Pork scaloppini with fresh sautéed tomatoes and garlic, accompanied by broccoli and sweet potatoes.

Sara Moulton's Pork Scaloppini

3/4 pound pork tenderloin
2 tablespoons flour
1 teaspoon olive oil

Salt and freshly ground black pepper
2 teaspoons minced garlic
2 cups fresh diced tomatoes

COUNTDOWN

- Microwave potatoes and broccoli.
- Make pork scaloppini.

1. Remove visible fat from pork, and cut into 1-inch slices. Place slices between two pieces of plastic wrap and flatten with the bottom of a heavy pan or meat tenderizer.

2. Place flour on a plate. Dip pork slices into flour, making sure both sides are covered.

3. Heat oil in a large nonstick skillet over medium-high heat. Brown pork 1 minute; turn and brown second side 1 minute. Salt and pepper the cooked sides to taste. Transfer to a plate.

4. Add garlic and tomatoes to the skillet, and cook 3 minutes. Spoon tomatoes over pork and serve.

Preparation time: 10 minutes ● Servings: 2

Calories 274 ● Calories from Fat 58 ● Total Fat 6.5 g ● Saturated Fat 1.6 g ● Monounsaturated Fat 3.1 g ● Cholesterol 108 mg ● Sodium 101 mg ● Carbohydrate 15 g ● Dietary Fiber 2.8 g ● Sugars 4.8 g ● Protein 38.4 g

Exchanges: 1/2 starch, 1 vegetable, 5 lean meat

Broccoli and Sweet Potatoes

3/4 pound sweet potatoes, peeled and cut into 1- to 2-inch pieces
1 1/2 cups broccoli florets (1/4 pound)
2 teaspoons olive oil
Salt and freshly ground black pepper

1. Add potatoes and broccoli to a microwave-safe bowl. Cover and microwave on high 5 minutes.
2. Remove and add olive oil and salt and pepper to taste. Toss well and serve.

Preparation time: 10 minutes ● Servings: 2

Calories 202 ● Calories from Fat 43 ● Total Fat 4.8 g ● Saturated Fat 0.7 g ● Monounsaturated Fat 3.3 g ● Cholesterol 0 mg ● Sodium 109 mg ● Carbohydrate 37.3 g ● Dietary Fiber 5.1 g ● Sugars 7.1 g ● Protein 4.4 g

Exchanges: 2 starch, 1 vegetable, 1/2 fat

HELPFUL HINTS:

■ Any type of potato and vegetable can be substituted.

■ Minced garlic can be found in the produce section or condiment section of the supermarket.

■ Diced fresh tomatoes can be found in the produce section of the supermarket.

SHOPPING LIST

Meat
3/4 pound pork tenderloin

Produce
1 container fresh diced tomatoes
3/4 pound sweet potatoes
1/4 pound broccoli florets

Staples
Olive oil
Minced garlic
Flour
Salt
Black peppercorns

SOUTHWESTERN HONEY-GLAZED PORK WITH SALSA POTATO SALAD

This cumin-scented pork hints of the Southwest. Adding salsa to potato salad completes the meal. I like to use red potatoes for the salad. To help them absorb more of the dressing flavor, mix them into the dressing while they are still hot.

Southwestern Honey-Glazed Pork

3/4 pound pork tenderloin
1 teaspoon minced garlic
1 1/2 tablespoons honey

1 teaspoon ground cumin
1 tablespoon reduced-sodium soy sauce
Olive oil spray

COUNTDOWN

■ Start potatoes boiling.
■ Make pork dish.
■ Finish potatoes.

1. Remove visible fat from pork and butterfly it. Cut pork almost in half lengthwise, and open like a book. Do not cut all of the way through. Cut in half crosswise to make two portions.

2. Mix the garlic, honey, cumin, and soy sauce together. Set aside.

3. Heat a nonstick skillet over medium-high heat. Spray with olive oil spray. Add pork, cover with a lid, and cook 5 minutes; turn and cook 4 more minutes. Spoon glaze over the pork, and cook 30 seconds.

4. Transfer pork to dinner plates, and spoon sauce on top. A meat thermometer should read 160°F. Serve.

Preparation time: 15 minutes ● Servings: 2

Calories 257 ● Calories from Fat 46 ● Total Fat 5.1 g ● Saturated Fat 1.4 g ● Monounsaturated Fat 2.3 g ● Cholesterol 108 mg ● Sodium 362 mg ● Carbohydrate 15.4 g ● Dietary Fiber 0.3 g ● Sugars 13.1 g ● Protein 36.5 g

Exchanges: 1 carbohydrate, 5 lean meat

Salsa Potato Salad

1 pound red potatoes
2 tablespoons mayonnaise
3 tablespoons plain nonfat yogurt
1/2 cup tomato salsa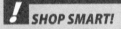
Salt and freshly ground black pepper

1. Wash potatoes, do not peel, and cut into 1-inch cubes.

2. *Microwave method*
   Place potatoes in a microwave-safe bowl, cover, and microwave 4 minutes on high.

2. *Stove-top method*
   Place in saucepan, and add cold water to cover. Bring water to a boil over high heat, cover with a lid, and simmer for 15 minutes or until cubes are cooked through.

3. Mix mayonnaise, yogurt, and salsa together in a serving bowl. Drain potatoes (if using stove-top method), and add to the serving bowl. Add salt and pepper to taste. Toss well, making sure potatoes are covered with sauce, and serve.

Preparation time: Microwave, 5 minutes; stove-top, 20 minutes ● Servings: 2

Calories 292 ● Calories from Fat 103 ● Total Fat 11.5 g ● Saturated Fat 1.6 g ● Monounsaturated Fat 2.5 g ● Cholesterol 5 mg ● Sodium 241 mg ● Carbohydrate 41.9 g ● Dietary Fiber 4.9 g ● Sugars 4.2 g ● Protein 6.6 g

Exchanges: 2 1/2 starch, 1 vegetable, 2 fat

HELPFUL HINTS:

■ Thin-cut boneless pork chops can be used instead of pork tenderloin.

■ Minced garlic can be found in jars in the produce or condiment sections of the supermarket.

SHOPPING LIST

Meat
3/4 pound pork tenderloin

Dairy
1 carton plain nonfat yogurt

Grocery
1 jar honey
1 bottle ground cumin
1 small bottle reduced-sodium soy sauce
1 jar tomato salsa

Produce
1 pound red potatoes

Staples
Minced garlic
Olive oil spray
Mayonnaise
Salt
Black peppercorns

SHOP SMART!

Salsa (per 2 tablespoons): 10 calories, 2 g carbohydrate, 65 mg sodium [*Example*: Newman's Own All-Natural Bandito Salsa]

WHISKEY PORK WITH ROSEMARY LENTILS

Whiskey lends a subtle, intriguing flavor to this pork dish. Brown sugar and mustard add a sweet and tangy finish.

The Rosemary Lentils calls for canned lentils, which work well here. Steamed lentils in a vacuum pack are available in some stores. These are not packed in sauce and have a firmer texture than canned ones. Try these lentils if your store carries them.

Whiskey Pork

2 6-ounce thin-cut boneless pork loin chops
   (1/2-inch thick)
Olive oil spray
1/4 cup whiskey

1/2 cup water
1 tablespoon brown sugar
1 tablespoon Dijon mustard

COUNTDOWN

■ Make pork chops.
■ Make lentils.

1. Remove visible fat from pork. Heat a nonstick skillet just big enough to fit the chops over medium-high heat. Spray with olive oil spray.
2. Add pork chops, and brown 2 minutes; turn and cook 1 more minute. Add whiskey. Cook 1 minute. Transfer to a plate. A meat thermometer should read 160°F.
3. Add water, sugar, and mustard to the skillet. Blend well, and raise the heat to high. Reduce to a smooth sauce, about 3 minutes. It will thicken as it reduces. Spoon sauce over chops and serve.

Preparation time: 10 minutes ● Servings: 2

Calories 269 ● Calories from Fat 72 ● Total Fat 8.0 g ● Saturated Fat 2.1 g ● Monounsaturated Fat 3.5 g ● Cholesterol 120 mg ● Sodium 185 mg ● Carbohydrate 7.6 g ● Dietary Fiber 0.3 g ● Sugars 6.8 g ● Protein 37.7 g

Exchanges: 1/2 carbohydrate, 5 lean meat

Rosemary Lentils

1/4 cup water
1 1/2 cups canned lentils, rinsed and drained ⚠
1 teaspoon minced garlic
1/2 teaspoon dried rosemary
Salt and freshly ground black pepper
2 tablespoons chopped fresh parsley (*optional*)

1. Place water, lentils, garlic, and rosemary in a saucepan. Bring to a boil, and cook 2–3 minutes.
2. Add salt and pepper to taste. Sprinkle with parsley (if desired) and serve.

Preparation time: 5 minutes ● Servings: 2

Calories 186 ● Calories from Fat 8 ● Total Fat 0.9 g ● Saturated Fat 0.2 g ● Monounsaturated Fat 0.2 g ● Cholesterol 0 mg ● Sodium 309 mg ● Carbohydrate 32.8 g ● Dietary Fiber 8.0 g ● Sugars 1.6 g ● Protein 12.3 g

Exchanges: 2 starch, 1 lean meat

HELPFUL HINTS:

■ Any type of pork chop can be used.

■ Any type of whiskey can be used.

■ Apple juice can be substituted for the whiskey.

■ Minced garlic can be found in jars in the produce or condiment sections of the supermarket.

SHOPPING LIST

Meat
2 6-ounce thin-cut boneless pork loin chops (1/2-inch thick)

Grocery
1 small bottle whiskey
1 package brown sugar
1 jar Dijon mustard
1 can lentils ⚠
1 bottle dried rosemary

Produce
1 bunch parsley (*optional*)

Staples
Olive oil spray
Minced garlic
Salt
Black peppercorns

⚠ **SHOP SMART!**

Canned lentils (per cup): 240 calories, 680 mg sodium

BEEF

Beef in Oyster Sauce with Chinese Noodles	200
Buffalo Cheeseburgers with Mixed Salad	202
Filet Marchand de Vin (Steak in Red Wine Sauce) with Sautéed Garlic Potatoes	204
Garlic Steak with Chili Pepper Potatoes	206
Honey-Mustard Crusted Steak with Garlic Rosemary Beans	208
Meatball, Beer, and Potato Stew	210
Mediterranean Steak with Minted Couscous	212
Mock Hungarian Goulash with Caraway Noodles	214
Pan-Fried Ropa Vieja (Flank Steak in Tomato Sauce) and Brown Rice	216
Pistachio-Crusted Beef and Vegetable Kabobs	218
Roast Beef Chopped Salad	220
Roast Beef Hash with Mixed Green Salad	222
Roast Beef Pita Pocket with Tomato and Onion Relish and Greek Summer Salad	224
Spaghetti Bolognese (Spaghetti and Meat Sauce) with Herbed Zucchini	226
Steak and Portobello Sandwich with Tapenade-Topped Tomatoes	228
Walnut-Crusted Buffalo Steak with Tomato and Bean Salad	230
Vietnamese Hot and Spicy Stir-Fry Beef and Chinese Noodles with Snow Peas	232

BEEF IN OYSTER SAUCE WITH CHINESE NOODLES

Oyster sauce flavors stir-fried beef in this typical Chinese dish. It takes a few minutes to prepare the ingredients, but only 5 minutes to stir-fry them. Oyster sauce is a tasty condiment to have on hand. Use it to flavor meat, vegetables, and other stir-fry dishes.

Beef in Oyster Sauce

2 tablespoons oyster sauce 🔳
3 tablespoons water
1 tablespoon sesame oil
2 cups trimmed green beans, cut in half (1/2 pound)

1/2 pound bottom round steak, cut into strips (2 inches by 1/2 inch)
2 tablespoons broken walnuts
Salt and freshly ground black pepper

COUNTDOWN

- Place water for noodles on to boil.
- Make noodles.
- Assemble ingredients.
- Stir-fry beef.

1. Mix oyster sauce and water together in a bowl. Set aside.
2. Heat oil in a wok or skillet over high heat until smoking. Add the green beans. Stir-fry 3 minutes.
3. Add steak. Stir-fry 1 minute.
4. Add oyster sauce and walnuts. Toss 30 seconds. Add salt and pepper to taste. Remove.
5. Add drained Chinese Noodles (see next recipe) to wok. Toss 1 minute.
6. Divide noodles between two dinner plates. Serve beef, green beans, and sauce on top.

Preparation time: 10 minutes ● Servings: 2

Calories 312 ● Calories from Fat 162 ● Total Fat 18.0 g ● Saturated Fat 3.3 g ● Monounsaturated Fat 7.8 g ● Cholesterol 68 mg ● Sodium 571 mg ● Carbohydrate 10.8 g ● Dietary Fiber 4.3 g ● Sugars 1.7 g ● Protein 27.9 g

Exchanges: 1/2 carbohydrate, 1 vegetable, 3 lean meat, 2 1/2 fat

Chinese Noodles

1/4 pound steamed or fresh Chinese noodles
  (1 3/4 cups cooked noodles)
Salt and freshly ground black pepper

1. Bring a large saucepan filled with water to a boil over high heat. Add noodles.
2. Boil 1 minute, drain, and add salt and pepper to taste.
3. Add to wok after beef and vegetables have been removed.

Preparation time: 5 minutes ● Servings: 2

Calories 145 ● Calories from Fat 14 ● Total Fat 1.6 g ● Saturated Fat 0.3 g ● Monounsaturated Fat 0 g ● Cholesterol 36 mg ● Sodium 8 mg ● Carbohydrate 27.0 g ● Dietary Fiber 1.0 g ● Sugars 1.1 g ● Protein 5.3 g

Exchanges: 2 starch

HELPFUL HINTS:

■ Bottom round steak is sometimes called London broil.

■ Angel hair pasta can be used instead of Chinese noodles.

SHOPPING LIST

Meat
1/2 pound bottom round steak

Grocery
1 bottle oyster sauce ▌
1 bottle sesame oil
1 small package broken walnuts

Produce
1/2 pound trimmed green beans
1/4 pound steamed or fresh Chinese noodles

Staples
Salt
Black peppercorns

▌ SHOP SMART!

Oyster sauce (per tablespoon): 9 calories, 492 mg sodium

BUFFALO CHEESEBURGERS WITH MIXED SALAD

Ground buffalo (also called ground bison) adds a new dimension to this all-American cheeseburger. Buffalo meat is very low in saturated fat and has a wonderful flavor. It can be found in many supermarkets, either fresh or frozen, and is worth looking for.

Buffalo Cheeseburgers

3/4 pound ground buffalo
1/4 cup frozen chopped onion, thawed
1 teaspoon minced garlic
Salt and freshly ground black pepper

2 teaspoons olive oil
4 slices whole-wheat bread
2 slices reduced-fat Cheddar cheese (2 ounces) 🔳

COUNTDOWN

■ Assemble salad.
■ Make buffalo burgers.

1. Combine buffalo, onion, garlic, and salt and pepper to taste in a medium bowl. Mix until combined. Form into two thin patties, each about 1/2-inch thick.
2. Drizzle oil on one side of each slice of bread.
3. Heat a large nonstick skillet over medium-high heat. Cook the burgers 3 minutes, turn, and cook 3 more minutes. Transfer to a plate.
4. In the same skillet, add two slices of bread, oiled side down. Top each with a slice of cheese and a burger. Cover the burgers with remaining slices of bread, oiled side up. Cook each sandwich 2 minutes, turn, and cook 2 more minutes or until golden brown. Remove to two dinner plates and serve with salad.

Preparation time: 15 minutes ● Servings: 2

Calories 425 ● Calories from Fat 104 ● Total Fat 11.5 g ● Saturated Fat 3.5 g ● Monounsaturated Fat 6.0 g ● Cholesterol 114 mg ● Sodium 530 mg ● Carbohydrate 26.5 g ● Dietary Fiber 4.2 g ● Sugars 4.2 g ● Protein 51.4 g

Exchanges: 2 starch, 1/2 vegetable, 4 lean meat, 1 fat

Mixed Salad

4 cups washed ready-to-eat mixed salad
2 tablespoons reduced-fat oil and vinegar dressing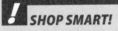

1. Place salad in a bowl, and toss with dressing. Serve.

Preparation time: 5 minutes ● Servings: 2

Calories 27 ● Calories from Fat 11 ● Total Fat 1.2 g ● Saturated Fat 0.1 g
● Monounsaturated Fat 0.3 g ● Cholesterol 1 mg ● Sodium 12 mg ●
Carbohydrate 3.8 g ● Dietary Fiber 2.0 g ● Sugars 1.8 g ● Protein 1.2 g

Exchanges: 1 vegetable

HELPFUL HINTS:

■ To quickly defrost frozen chopped onion, place in a strainer and run hot tap water over the onion.

■ Shape the burgers to fit the sliced bread.

SHOPPING LIST

Beef
3/4 pound ground buffalo

Dairy
1 package reduced-fat Cheddar cheese

Grocery
1 package frozen chopped onion

Produce
1 bag washed ready-to-eat mixed salad

Staples
Olive oil
Minced garlic
Reduced-fat oil and vinegar dressing
Whole-wheat bread
Salt
Black peppercorns

SHOP SMART!

Low-fat Cheddar cheese (per ounce): 49 calories, 2.0 g fat, 1.2 g saturated fat, 174 mg sodium.

Reduced-fat vinaigrette or oil and vinegar dressing (per tablespoon): 11 calories, 1.0 g fat, 4 mg sodium

FILET MARCHAND DE VIN (STEAK IN RED WINE SAUCE) WITH SAUTÉED GARLIC POTATOES

This traditional French bistro steak, cooked in a red wine sauce, is easy to make and elegant enough for company.

Filet Marchand de Vin (Steak in Red Wine Sauce)

Olive oil spray
1/2 pound beef tenderloin steak, about 3/4-inch thick
1/2 cup fresh diced onion
3/4 cup sliced mushrooms (2 ounces)
1 tablespoon flour
1/2 cup dry red wine

1/4 cup fat-free low-sodium chicken broth
1 tablespoon ketchup
1 teaspoon dried thyme
Salt and freshly ground black pepper
2 tablespoons freshly chopped parsley (*optional*)

COUNTDOWN

- Start potatoes.
- Make steak.
- Finish potatoes.

1. Spray a medium nonstick skillet with olive oil spray. Remove visible fat from steak.
2. Heat skillet over medium-high heat. Brown the steak 1 minute; turn over and brown 1 more minute.
3. Lower heat to medium, and add onion and mushrooms. Cook for 2 minutes. Cook 1 more minute if you prefer meat more well-done. A meat thermometer should read 145°F for medium-rare and 160°F for medium.
4. Transfer steak to individual plates.
5. Add flour to the skillet, and mix with the vegetables until dissolved.
6. Raise the heat to high, and add wine. Cook 1 minute. Add the broth, ketchup, and thyme. Cook 2–3 minutes to reduce liquid and thicken.
7. Add salt and pepper to taste. Divide steak and potatoes between two dinner plates. Spoon sauce over steak and potatoes; sprinkle with parsley (if desired) and serve.

Preparation time: 15 minutes ● Servings: 2

Calories 285 ● Calories from Fat 82 ● Total Fat 9.1 g ● Saturated Fat 3.0 g ● Monounsaturated Fat 4.0g ● Cholesterol 72 mg ● Sodium 223 mg ● Carbohydrate 12.2 g ● Dietary Fiber 1.4 g ● Sugars 2.1 g ● Protein 27.5 g

Exchanges: 2 vegetable, 4 lean meat, 1 fat

Sautéed Garlic Potatoes

1 pound canned potatoes, sliced, rinsed, and drained (about 3 cups)
2 teaspoons minced garlic
1/2 cup fat-free low-sodium chicken broth
2 teaspoons olive oil
Salt and freshly ground black pepper

Microwave method
1. Place potatoes, garlic, and chicken broth in a microwave-safe bowl. Microwave on high 2 minutes or until potatoes are warmed.

2. Add olive oil and salt and pepper to taste. Gently toss together.

Stove-top method
1. Place potatoes, garlic, and chicken broth in a saucepan over medium-high heat. Cook 3–4 minutes or until potatoes are warmed through.

2. Add olive oil and salt and pepper to taste. Gently toss together.

Preparation time: 5 minutes ● Servings: 2

Calories 188 ● Calories from Fat 45 ● Total Fat 5.0 g ● Saturated Fat 0.7 g ● Monounsaturated Fat 3.3 g ● Cholesterol 0 mg ● Sodium 156 mg ● Carbohydrate 32.2 g ● Dietary Fiber 5.5 g ● Sugars 1.4 g ● Protein 4.2 g

Exchanges: 2 starch, 1 fat

HELPFUL HINTS:

■ Any type of red wine can be used.

■ Diced fresh onions can be found in the produce section of the supermarket.

SHOPPING LIST

Meat
1/2 pound beef tenderloin steak, about 3/4-inch thick

Grocery
1 bottle dry red wine
1 can fat-free low-sodium chicken broth
1 small bottle ketchup
1 bottle dried thyme
2 14.5-ounce cans sliced potatoes

Produce
1 container fresh diced onions
1 container sliced mushrooms (2 ounces needed)
1 bunch parsley (*optional*)

Staples
Olive oil spray
Olive oil
Flour
Minced garlic
Salt
Black peppercorns

GARLIC STEAK WITH CHILI PEPPER POTATOES

Garlic plays an important role in this steak and potatoes dinner. Garlic has been praised for its many health benefits and its flavor. Garlic is low in calories, and when cooked slowly without browning, it develops a mellow and nut-like flavor.

Poblano pepper is used in this recipe. Any type of pepper can be used. Serrano peppers (very hot when fresh) or jalapeño peppers will work well.

Garlic Steak

1/2 pound tenderloin steak (about 3/4-inch thick)
Olive oil spray
Salt and freshly ground black pepper

3 teaspoons minced garlic
1 cup fresh diced onion
1/4 pound sliced button mushrooms (about 1 2/3 cups)

COUNTDOWN

■ Start potatoes.
■ Cook steak.
■ Finish potatoes.

1. Remove visible fat from the steak. Heat a nonstick skillet over medium-high heat, and spray with olive oil spray. Add the steak, and brown 1 minute. Sprinkle with salt and pepper to taste. Turn and brown second side 1 more minute.

2. Lower heat to medium. Add garlic, onion, and mushrooms. Continue to sauté the steak for 3 minutes for a 3/4-inch thick steak. A meat thermometer should read 145°F for medium-rare. Cook longer for more well-done meat. Transfer to a dish.

3. Continue to cook onion and mushrooms for 2 more minutes. Divide between two dinner plates, place steak on top, and serve.

Preparation time: 10 minutes ● Servings: 2

Calories 253 ● Calories from Fat 82 ● Total Fat 9.1 g ● Saturated Fat 3.0 g ● Monounsaturated Fat 3.8 g ● Cholesterol 72 mg ● Sodium 123 mg ● Carbohydrate 14.8 g ● Dietary Fiber 3.6 g ● Sugars 3.7 g ● Protein 30.1 g

Exchanges: 3 vegetable, 3 lean meat, 1 fat

Chili Pepper Potatoes

1 pound red potatoes, washed and cut into 1/2-inch pieces
   (about 2 3/4 cups)
4 cups washed ready-to-eat spinach
2 teaspoons olive oil
1/2 cup coarsely chopped poblano pepper (stem and seeds removed)
Salt and freshly ground black pepper

1. Place the potatoes in a medium saucepan, and cover with cold water. Cover pan with a lid, and bring to a boil over high heat.

2. Boil for 10 minutes or until the potatoes are soft.

3. Add spinach to the saucepan.

4. Transfer 2 tablespoons water to a bowl. Add olive oil and poblano pepper to the bowl.

5. Drain potatoes and spinach, and add to the bowl.

6. Add salt and pepper to taste. Toss well and serve.

Preparation time: 15 minutes ● Servings: 2

Calories 204 ● Calories from Fat 43.6 ● Total Fat 4.9 g ● Saturated Fat 0.7 g ● Monounsaturated Fat 3.3 g ● Cholesterol 0 mg ● Sodium 14 mg ● Carbohydrate 37.2 g ● Dietary Fiber 3.9 g ● Sugars 2.3 g ● Protein 4.5 g

Exchanges: 2 starch, 1 vegetable, 1/2 fat

HELPFUL HINTS:

■ Diced fresh onions can be found in the produce section of the supermarket.

■ The steak can be grilled or broiled instead of sautéed.

HONEY-MUSTARD CRUSTED STEAK WITH GARLIC ROSEMARY BEANS

Honey mustard and cumin create a tangy topping for grass-fed strip steak. Garlic and rosemary-flavored cannellini beans complete this quick dinner.

Honey-Mustard Crusted Steak

Olive oil spray

2 tablespoons honey mustard 🔲

1 teaspoon ground cumin

3/4 pound grass-fed strip steak, visible fat removed

Salt and freshly ground black pepper

COUNTDOWN

■ Preheat broiler.
■ Prepare ingredients.
■ Start steak.
■ Make beans.
■ Finish steak.

1. Preheat broiler. Line a baking tray with foil, and spray with olive oil spray.

2. Mix honey mustard and cumin together in a bowl.

3. Place steak on foil, and broil 5 inches from heat for 3 minutes; turn and spread mustard mixture over steak.

4. Broil 4 minutes. A meat thermometer should read 145°F for medium-rare.

5. Transfer to two dinner plates, sprinkle with salt and pepper to taste, and serve.

Preparation time: 15 minutes ● Servings: 2

Calories 246 ● Calories from Fat 56 ● Total Fat 6.2 g ● Saturated Fat 2.0 g ● Monounsaturated Fat 2.8 g ● Cholesterol 96 mg ● Sodium 115 mg ● Carbohydrate 3.9 g ● Dietary Fiber 0.1 g ● Sugars 3.0 g ● Protein 39.5 g

Exchange: 5 lean meat

Garlic Rosemary Beans

1 1/2 cups cannellini beans (or navy beans), rinsed and drained
1/4 cup fat-free low-sodium chicken broth
1 teaspoon minced garlic
1 teaspoon dried rosemary
Salt and freshly ground black pepper

1. Place beans in a saucepan, and heat over medium heat.

2. Add chicken broth, garlic, and rosemary. Simmer 3 minutes.

3. Add salt and pepper to taste and serve.

Preparation time: 5 minutes ● Servings: 2

Calories 236 ● Calories from Fat 9.4 ● Total Fat 1.1 g ● Saturated Fat 0.4 g
● Monounsaturated Fat 0.1 g ● Cholesterol 0 mg ● Sodium 78 mg ●
Carbohydrate 43.5 g ● Dietary Fiber 10.4 g ● Sugars 0.6 g ● Protein 15.1 g

Exchanges: 2 1/2 starch, 1 lean meat

HELPFUL HINTS:

■ If grass-fed strip steak is not available, use 1/2 pound beef tenderloin.

■ Honey mustard can be found with the other mustards in the condiment aisle.

■ Any type of beans, such as red kidney beans, can be used instead of cannellini beans.

SHOPPING LIST

Meat
3/4 pound grass-fed strip steak

Grocery
1 jar honey mustard ⚠
1 bottle ground cumin
1 can cannellini beans (or navy beans)
1 bottle dried rosemary

Staples
Olive oil spray
Fat-free low-sodium chicken broth
Minced garlic
Salt
Black peppercorns

⚠ SHOP SMART!

Honey mustard (per tablespoon): 30 calories, 0 fat, 15 mg sodium [*Example*: Grey Poupon]

MEATBALL, BEER, AND POTATO STEW

Fennel-flavored meatballs, apples, and beer mingle in make this quick casserole/soup. The beer adds an intriguing depth of flavor. This is a simple one-pot meal where all of the ingredients are placed in a large pot and left to cook on their own. This dinner will freeze well. If you have time, make double and save half for another quick meal.

Meatball, Beer, and Potato Stew

1/2 tablespoon fennel seeds
1/2 pound 95% lean ground beef
Salt and freshly ground black pepper
2 teaspoons olive oil
1 cup fresh diced onion
1 cup fresh diced green bell pepper

1 cup fresh sliced Granny Smith apples
3 cups sliced tomatoes
8 ounces beer
1 cup fat-free low-sodium chicken broth
1 teaspoon dried thyme
1 cup canned sweet potatoes, rinsed and drained (1/2 pound)

COUNTDOWN

■ Prepare all of the ingredients.
■ Make stew.

1. Mix fennel seeds into ground beef. Add salt and pepper to taste. Make into 1- to 2-inch meatballs (about 8 meatballs).

2. Heat olive oil in a large nonstick casserole over medium-high heat. Add meatballs, onion, and green pepper. Sauté 5 minutes, turning meatballs over several times to brown on all sides.

3. Add the apples, tomatoes, beer, chicken broth, and thyme. Bring to simmer, cover with a lid, and simmer gently 5 minutes.

4. Add sweet potatoes, and simmer 2 minutes. Ladle soup into two bowls and serve.

Preparation time: 15 minutes ● Servings: 2

Calories 498 ● Calories from Fat 107 ● Total Fat 11.9 g ● Saturated Fat 3.5 g ● Monounsaturated Fat 6.0 g ● Cholesterol 144 mg ● Sodium 424 mg ● Carbohydrate 61.4 g ● Dietary Fiber 11.4 g ● Sugars 24.3 g ● Protein 32.3 g

Exchanges: 2 starch, 1/2 fruit, 2 vegetable, 1/2 carbohydrate, 4 lean meat, 1 fat

HELPFUL HINTS:

■ Any type of beer can be used. The alcohol burns off in the cooking.

■ When using dried spices, make sure the bottle is no more than 6 months old.

■ Diced fresh onions and green bell pepper can be found in the produce section of the supermarket.

■ Fresh sliced apples can be found in the produce section of the supermarket.

 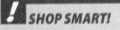

MEDITERRANEAN STEAK WITH MINTED COUSCOUS

Enjoy this sautéed steak flavored with the bounty of the Mediterranean—olives, walnuts, and capers—in just 15 minutes.

Precooked, packaged couscous takes only 5 minutes to make. It's made from semolina flour and is, in fact, a form of pasta rather than what many people think is a grain. You just boil water, remove from heat, add the couscous, cover, and let stand. In this case I've added fresh mint and chopped tomatoes to add a fresh flavor that goes well with the steak.

Mediterranean Steak

1/2 pound beef tenderloin steak (3/4-inch thick)
Pinch cayenne pepper (about 1/8 teaspoon)
Olive oil spray

1 tablespoon walnut pieces
8 sliced pimento-stuffed green olives
Salt and freshly ground black pepper

COUNTDOWN

- Bring water for couscous to a boil.
- Prepare ingredients for steak.
- Make couscous.
- Finish steak.

1. Remove visible fat from steak. Sprinkle with cayenne.
2. Heat a small nonstick skillet over medium-high heat. Spray with olive oil spray, and add steak. Brown steak 1 minute; turn and brown 1 more minute.
3. Sprinkle walnuts and olives into skillet and over steak. Lower heat to medium, and cook 2 minutes for medium-rare. A meat thermometer should read 145°F. Cook 2 minutes longer for thick steak. Add salt and pepper to taste.
4. To serve, place couscous on two dinner plates, slice steak, and place steak on top. Spoon pan juices over steak.

Preparation time: 10 minutes ● Servings: 2

Calories 227 ● Calories from Fat 116 ● Total Fat 12.9 g ● Saturated Fat 3.4 g ● Monounsaturated Fat 5.5 g ● Cholesterol 72 mg ● Sodium 246 mg ● Carbohydrate 1.4 g ● Dietary Fiber 0.7 g ● Sugars 0.1 g ● Protein 25.8 g

Exchanges: 4 lean meat, 1 fat

Minted Couscous

1 cup water
1/2 cup whole-wheat couscous
1 cup fresh diced tomatoes
1/4 cup chopped fresh mint
Salt and freshly ground black pepper

1. Bring water to a boil over high heat. Remove from heat. Add couscous and tomatoes. Cover with a lid, and let stand 5 minutes. When ready, fluff up with a fork.
2. Add mint and salt and pepper to taste.

Preparation time: 10 minutes ● Servings: 2

Calories 179 ● Calories from Fat 4 ● Total Fat 0.5 g ● Saturated Fat 0.1 g ● Monounsaturated Fat 0.1 g ● Cholesterol 0 mg ● Sodium 9 mg ● Carbohydrate 37.0 g ● Dietary Fiber 3.3 g ● Sugars 2.4 g ● Protein 6.3 g

Exchanges: 2 starch, 1 vegetable

HELPFUL HINTS:

■ Diced fresh tomatoes can be found in the produce section of the supermarket.

■ Use a skillet that just fits the steak to capture the pan juices. A larger skillet will cause the juices to boil off.

SHOPPING LIST

Meat
1/2 pound beef tenderloin steak

Grocery
1 small bottle cayenne pepper
1 small package walnut pieces
1 bottle pimento-stuffed green olives
1 box whole-wheat couscous

Produce
1 container fresh diced tomatoes
1 bunch mint

Staples
Olive oil spray
Salt
Black peppercorns

MOCK HUNGARIAN GOULASH WITH CARAWAY NOODLES

An exquisite tomato sauce flavored with onion, green pepper, and paprika, dressing a cut of succulent beef, is the foundation for Hungarian goulash. Here's a quick version. The secret to a good Hungarian goulash is good Hungarian paprika. Paprika is the Hungarian name for both sweet pepper and the powder made from it. Ordinary paprika comes in varying degrees of flavor, from pungent to virtually tasteless. True Hungarian paprika may be hot or mild and can be found in most supermarkets.

Mock Hungarian Goulash

Olive oil spray
1/2 cup frozen chopped onion
1 cup frozen chopped green bell pepper
2 cups sliced Portobello mushrooms
1 tablespoon Hungarian paprika or 1 1/2 tablespoons ordinary paprika
1/2 cup low-sodium pasta sauce 🚺

1/2 cup water
6 ounces thick-sliced lean deli roast beef, cut into 1/2-inch slices 🚺
Salt and freshly ground black pepper
2 tablespoons nonfat sour cream
2 medium tomatoes, cut into wedges

COUNTDOWN

■ Place water for noodles on to boil.
■ Make goulash.
■ Boil pasta.

1. Heat a nonstick skillet over medium-high heat. Spray with olive oil spray. Add onion, green pepper, and mushrooms. Sauté 1 minute.
2. Sprinkle paprika over vegetables, and sauté 2 minutes.
3. Add pasta sauce and water. Simmer 1 minute.
4. Remove from heat. Add roast beef and salt and pepper to taste.
5. Serve over noodles. Dot the goulash with sour cream. Arrange tomatoes on the side.

Preparation time: 10 minutes ● Servings: 2

Calories 301 ● Calories from Fat 81 ● Total Fat 9.0 g ● Saturated Fat 3.1 g ● Monounsaturated Fat 3.7 g ● Cholesterol 46 mg ● Sodium 99 mg ● Carbohydrate 27.8 g ● Dietary Fiber 7.4 g ● Sugars 13.9 g ● Protein 27.7 g

Exchanges: 1/2 starch, 3 vegetable, 3 lean meat, 1 fat

Caraway Noodles

3 ounces flat egg noodles (about 1 1/2 cups)
1 teaspoon olive oil
2 teaspoons caraway seeds
Salt and freshly ground black pepper

1. Bring a large pot with 2–3 quarts of water to a boil over high heat. Add the noodles. Boil 3–4 minutes or according to package instructions.

2. Drain, leaving about 2 tablespoons water on the noodles.

3. Add olive oil and caraway seeds and salt and pepper to taste to noodles. Toss and serve.

Preparation time: 10 minutes ● Servings: 2

Calories 185 ● Calories from Fat 29 ● Total Fat 3.2 g ● Saturated Fat 0.4 g ● Monounsaturated Fat 1.9 g ● Cholesterol 0 mg ● Sodium 2 mg ● Carbohydrate 33.0 g ● Dietary Fiber 2.2 g ● Sugars 1.1 g ● Protein 6.0 g

Exchanges: 2 starch, 1/2 fat

HELPFUL HINTS:

■ Ask for the roast beef to be cut into a 1/2-inch-thick slice. It is easier to cut into cubes.

■ The roast beef will be heated in the sauce. To prevent overcooking the beef, buy rare roast beef.

■ Any type of pasta can be used.

SHOPPING LIST

Deli
6 ounces thick-sliced lean deli roast beef, cut into 1/2-inch slices ▉

Dairy
1 carton nonfat sour cream

Grocery
1 package frozen/chopped onion
1 package frozen/chopped green pepper
1 container Hungarian paprika
1 bottle low-sodium pasta sauce ▉
1 small package flat egg noodles
1 bottle caraway seeds

Produce
1 container sliced Portobello mushrooms
2 medium tomatoes

Staples
Olive oil
Olive oil spray
Salt
Black peppercorns

▉ **SHOP SMART!**

Oven-roasted, no-salt-added, choice roast beef (per ounce): 45 calories, 1.7 g fat, 0.75 g saturated fat, 20 mg sodium
[*Example*: Boars Head brand]

Low-sodium pasta sauce (per 1/2 cup): 112 calories, 3.5 g fat, 17.7 g carbohydrate, 39 mg sodium

PAN-FRIED ROPA VIEJA (FLANK STEAK IN TOMATO SAUCE) AND BROWN RICE

"Old cloths" is the literal translation of *ropa vieja*. This Cuban dish is made with leftover meat or flank steak that has been simmered for several hours, until it falls apart into strings. Ropa Vieja can be made with any shredded meat that has been boiled or fried. As long as it is cooked with a traditional sauce of onions, garlic, green peppers, and tomatoes, it's Ropa Vieja.

For this quick version, I cut the steak into paper-thin slices and sautéed it first. Then I added it to the sauce for a few minutes so the steak can absorb the flavors from the sauce. The result is a dish that takes a fraction of the time to prepare but still has the feeling and flavor of the traditional long-cooked dish.

Pan-Fried Ropa Vieja (Flank Steak in Tomato Sauce)

1/2 pound beef tenderloin steak
Olive oil spray
1 cup fresh diced onion
1 cup thinly sliced carrots
1 teaspoon minced garlic crushed
1 cup fresh diced green bell pepper

1 3/4 cups canned low-sodium whole tomatoes, with juice
1 teaspoon dried oregano
1/2 cup drained, sliced pimentos
Salt and freshly ground black pepper

COUNTDOWN

■ Make rice.
■ While rice cooks, prepare and cook meat dish.

1. Cut meat with the grain, into paper-thin slices.
2. Heat a medium nonstick skillet over medium-high heat. Spray with olive oil spray.
3. Sauté meat for about 2 minutes, turning brown all sides. Transfer to a plate. Reduce heat to medium.
4. In same pan, sauté onion and carrots 3 minutes. Add garlic and green pepper, and continue to sauté for 5 more minutes, stirring as they cook.
5. Add whole tomatoes and oregano. Using a spoon, break up whole tomatoes as they cook. Simmer 5 minutes.
6. Return meat to the pan. Mix well. Add pimentos and salt and pepper to taste. Cook 1 minute. Serve over rice.

Preparation time: 20 minutes ● Servings: 2

Calories 301 ● Calories from Fat 81 ● Total Fat 9.0 g ● Saturated Fat 3.1 g ● Monounsaturated Fat 3.6 g ● Cholesterol 72 mg ● Sodium 137mg ● Carbohydrate 28.5 g ● Dietary Fiber 7.5 g ● Sugars 14.1 g ● Protein 29.5 g

Exchanges: 5 vegetable, 3 lean meat, 1 fat

Brown Rice

1 package microwaveable brown rice (to measure 1 1/2 cups cooked)
Salt and freshly ground black pepper

1. Microwave rice according to package instructions, and measure out 1 1/2 cups cooked rice. Reserve remaining rice for another meal.
2. Add salt and pepper to taste. Serve with Ropa Vieja.

Preparation time: 5 minutes ● Servings: 2

Calories 180 ● Calories from Fat 23 ● Total Fat 2.6 g ● Saturated Fat 0.4 g ● Monounsaturated Fat 0.8 g ● Cholesterol 0 mg ● Sodium 11 mg ● Carbohydrate 29.3 g ● Dietary Fiber 1.5 g ● Sugars 0 g ● Protein 3.8 g

Exchanges: 2 starch

HELPFUL HINTS:

■ Any type of quick-cooking rice can be used in this recipe.

■ Diced fresh onions and green bell pepper can be found in the produce section of the supermarket.

SHOPPING LIST

Meat
1/2 pound beef tenderloin steak

Grocery
1 large can low-sodium whole tomatoes 🛈
1 bottle dried oregano
1 bottle or can sliced pimentos
1 package microwaveable brown rice

Produce
1 container fresh diced onion
1 container fresh diced green bell pepper
1 container sliced carrots

Staples
Olive oil spray
Minced garlic
Salt
Black peppercorns

🛈 SHOP SMART!

Low-sodium canned whole tomatoes (per cup): 41 calories, 0.3 g fat, 9.6 g carbohydrate, 24 mg sodium

PISTACHIO-CRUSTED BEEF AND VEGETABLE KABOBS

Pistachios and hot pepper jelly coat juicy beef cubes for this spicy, crunchy barbecue dinner. To make this a quick and easy dinner, ask the butcher to cut the beef into cubes for kabobs before you take it home. Mushrooms, red bell pepper, and corn-on-the-cob complete this meal.

Pistachio-Crusted Beef and Mixed Vegetable Kabobs

2 tablespoons hot pepper jam or jelly, divided
2 tablespoons finely chopped, unsalted pistachios
1/2 pound beef tenderloin steak, fat removed and cut into 1 1/2- to 2-inch cubes
2 cups red bell pepper, cut into 1-inch pieces

2 cups baby bello mushrooms, cut into 1-inch pieces
Olive oil spray
2 medium ears corn-on-the-cob, husked
4 skewers

COUNTDOWN

■ Prepare the ingredients.
■ Heat the grill.
■ Make the kabobs and corn.

1. Place 1 tablespoon jam in a bowl, and add the pistachios. Stir. Roll meat in jam and nuts.
2. Thread meat, red bell pepper, and mushrooms onto the skewers. Spray with olive oil spray.
3. Place corn on a large piece of foil. Spread remaining 1 tablespoon jam on corn. Close foil to seal the corn.
4. Grill skewers for 5 minutes; turn and grill 3 more minutes for medium-rare. A meat thermometer should read 145°F. Grill 2 more minutes for more well-done meat. A meat thermometer should read 165°F.
5. At the same time, place corn on the grill. Grill 5 minutes, turn, and grill 5 more minutes.

Preparation time: 15 minutes ● Servings: 2

Calories 467 ● Calories from Fat 134 ● Total Fat 14.9 g ● Saturated Fat 3.9 g ● Monounsaturated Fat 6.3g ● Cholesterol 72 mg ● Sodium 101 mg ● Carbohydrate 54.0 g ● Dietary Fiber 7.6 g ● Sugars 16.1 g ● Protein 35.4 g

Exchanges: 1 1/2 starch, 2 vegetable, 1 carbohydrate, 4 lean meat, 1 fat

HELPFUL HINTS:

■ Green or yellow bell pepper can be used instead of red bell pepper.

■ Any type of mushroom can be used.

■ To help the cubes of meat cook evenly on a skewer, leave about 1/4 inch of space between them when you thread them on the skewers. This allows the heat to reach the sides of the food as well as the top and bottom.

■ Chop the pistachios in a food processor.

■ A stove-top grill or broiler can be used for this dinner.

SHOPPING LIST

Meat
1/2 pound beef tenderloin steak

Grocery
1 jar hot pepper jam or jelly
1 container unsalted pistachios

Produce
1 large red bell pepper
1 container baby bello mushrooms
2 medium ears corn-on-the-cob

Staples
Olive oil spray
4 skewers

ROAST BEEF CHOPPED SALAD

This colorful, light dinner combines cubes of vegetables with roast beef. The secret is to cut all of the ingredients into small 1/2-inch cubes. Every bite will contain different flavor combinations. Using roast beef from the deli section of the market makes this meal a breeze. Be sure to buy low-sodium roast beef. Ask for it to be cut into a 1/2-inch-thick slice. Then, it can easily be cut into cubes.

Roast Beef Chopped Salad

1 cup celery, sliced into 1/2-inch pieces
1 cup green bell pepper, cut into 1/2-inch pieces
1 cup peeled carrots, sliced 1/2-inch pieces
4 cups romaine lettuce leaves, sliced into
    1/2-inch pieces

6 ounces deli roast beef, thick-sliced, cut into
    1/2-inch cubes ⚡
2 crusty whole-grain rolls (2 ounces each)
3 tablespoons reduced-fat oil and vinegar dressing ⚡
2 scallions, sliced
2 teaspoons olive oil

COUNTDOWN

■ Preheat oven to 350°F for the rolls.
■ Prepare ingredients.
■ Assemble salad.

1. Preheat oven to 350°F.

2. Prepare all of the salad vegetables and the roast beef, using 1/2-inch pieces as a guideline. They should all be about the same size.

3. Place rolls in oven to warm, 5 minutes.

4. Place celery, green pepper, carrots, and lettuce in a medium bowl. Add dressing and toss. Add roast beef and scallions, and toss again.

5. Remove bread from oven, drizzle with olive oil, and serve with the salad.

Preparation time: 10 minutes ● Servings: 2

Calories 407 ● Calories from Fat 128 ● Total Fat 14.2 g ● Saturated Fat 3.6 g ● Monounsaturated Fat 6.7 g ● Cholesterol 47 mg ● Sodium 425 mg ● Carbohydrate 44.2 g ● Dietary Fiber 10.2 g ● Sugars 12.6 g ● Protein 28.9 g

Exchanges: 2 starch, 2 vegetable, 3 lean meat, 1 1/2 fat

HELPFUL HINTS:

■ Any type of lean, low-sodium roasted meat can be used in the salad.

■ Rolls can be warmed in a toaster oven.

SHOPPING LIST

Meat
1/2 pound deli roast beef, thick-sliced, 1/2-inch slices *!*

Grocery
2 crusty whole-grain rolls

Produce
1 small bunch celery
1 green bell pepper
1 container peeled carrots
1 small head romaine lettuce
1 bunch scallions

Staples
Reduced-fat oil and vinegar dressing *!*
Olive oil

! SHOP SMART!

Oven-roasted, no-salt-added, choice roast beef (per ounce): 45 calories, 1.7 g fat, 0.75 g saturated fat, 20 mg sodium
[*Example*: Boars Head brand]

Reduced-fat vinaigrette or oil and vinegar dressing (per tablespoon): 11 calories, 1.0 g fat, 4 mg sodium

ROAST BEEF HASH WITH MIXED GREEN SALAD

Roast beef, shiitake mushrooms, and fresh thyme transform a '50s-style hash into a speedy modern meal. This hash keeps well. Make a double batch, if you have time.

Roast Beef Hash

2 teaspoons olive oil
1 pound canned potatoes, rinsed and drained
   (about 2 3/4 cups)
1 cup fresh diced onion
1 1/2 cups shiitake mushrooms, sliced (3 1/2 ounces)
1 tablespoon pine nuts
6 ounces lean deli roast beef, thick-sliced,
   cut into 1/2-inch cubes ⚡

1 cup sliced canned sweet pimento, drained
1 teaspoon dried thyme
2 tablespoons flour
1/2 cup fat-free low-sodium chicken broth
1/2 cup water
Salt and freshly ground black pepper

COUNTDOWN

■ Make hash.
■ While hash cooks, make salad.

1. Heat oil in a nonstick skillet over medium-high heat. Add potatoes, onion, and mushrooms. Sauté 5 minutes.

2. Add pine nuts, roast beef, pimento, and thyme. Stir for 2 minutes.

3. Push ingredients to the sides of the skillet, leaving a hole in the center. Add the flour and then broth and water. Stir until sauce thickens. Toss with the ingredients. The sauce will lightly bind the hash together.

4. Add salt and pepper to taste and serve.

Preparation time: 10 minutes ● Servings: 2

Calories 435 ● Calories from Fat 115 ● Total Fat 12.8 g ● Saturated Fat 3.5 g ● Monounsaturated Fat 6.4 g ● Cholesterol 45 mg ● Sodium 234 mg ● Carbohydrate 51.3 g ● Dietary Fiber 9.6 g ● Sugars 7.3 g ● Protein 30.3 g

Exchanges: 2 1/2 starch, 2 vegetable, 3 lean meat, 1 fat

Mixed Green Salad

4 cups washed ready-to-eat mixed salad
2 tablespoons reduced-fat oil and vinegar salad dressing ⚠

1. Toss salad with dressing and serve.

Preparation time: 5 minutes ● Servings: 2

Calories 27 ● Calories from Fat 11 ● Total Fat 1.2 g ● Saturated Fat 0.1 g ● Monounsaturated Fat 0.3 g ● Cholesterol 1 mg ● Sodium 12 mg ● Carbohydrate 3.8 g ● Dietary Fiber 2.0 g ● Sugars 1.8 g ● Protein 1.2

Exchanges: 1 vegetable

HELPFUL HINTS:

■ Ask the deli to cut the roast beef into a 1/2-inch-thick slice. It can then easily be cut into cubes.

■ Any type of canned beans can be used in the salad.

■ Diced fresh onions can be found in the produce section of the supermarket.

SHOPPING LIST

Deli
6 ounces thick-sliced lean deli roast beef, cut into a 1/2-inch-thick slices ⚠

Grocery
1 large can sliced potatoes
1 package pine nuts
1 bottle dried thyme
1 can/jar sliced sweet pimento

Produce
1 container fresh diced onion
1 container shiitake mushrooms (3 1/2 ounces needed)
1 bag washed ready-to-eat mixed salad

Staples
Olive oil
Flour
Fat-free low-sodium chicken broth
Reduced-fat oil and vinegar salad dressing ⚠
Salt
Black peppercorns

⚠ SHOP SMART!

Oven-roasted, no-salt-added, choice roast beef (per ounce): 45 calories, 1.7 g fat, 0.75 g saturated fat, 20 mg sodium
Example: Boars Head brand

Reduced-fat vinaigrette or oil and vinegar dressing (per tablespoon): 11 calories, 1.0 g fat, 4 mg sodium

ROAST BEEF PITA POCKET WITH TOMATO AND ONION RELISH AND GREEK SUMMER SALAD

Here's a cool combination for a warm summer evening or just a quick sandwich supper. Tomato and onion are mixed together to make a tangy, uncooked relish that delivers a refreshing texture and flavor. When combined, the relish and roast beef turn ordinary pita pockets into a tasty, colorful meal.

Look for large pita bread. I find that whole-wheat pita bread has more texture and flavor than plain. If you can only find small pitas, use two per serving.

Roast Beef Pita Pocket with Tomato and Onion Relish

1 cup fresh diced tomato

1 tablespoon fresh diced onion

1 tablespoon balsamic vinegar

3 tablespoons fresh cilantro

Salt and freshly ground black pepper

2 large whole-wheat pita breads (6 1/2 inches each)

6 ounces sliced lean deli roast beef, cut into strips ⚡

COUNTDOWN

■ Prepare onion and tomato relish, and set aside to marinate a few minutes.

■ Make the Greek Summer Salad.

■ Complete the pita pockets.

1. Mix tomato, onion, balsamic vinegar, and cilantro together in a bowl. Add salt and pepper to taste.

2. Toast pita breads in a toaster oven to warm slightly. Do not let it get too crisp. Cut pita breads in half and open pockets. Spoon half of the relish into the pockets. Add the roast beef, and finish with the remaining relish. Serve.

Preparation time: 10 minutes ● Servings: 2

Calories 360 ● Calories from Fat 62 ● Total Fat 6.9 g ● Saturated Fat 2.6 g ● Monounsaturated Fat 2.5 g ● Cholesterol 45 mg ● Sodium 410 mg ● Carbohydrate 47.6 g ● Dietary Fiber 7.2 g ● Sugars 7.0 g ● Protein 29.0 g

Exchanges: 2 1/2 starch, 1 vegetable, 3 lean meat

Greek Summer Salad

1 teaspoon dried oregano

2 tablespoons reduced-fat vinaigrette dressing **/**

2 cups peeled, sliced cucumber

2 cups seeded, sliced green bell pepper

10 green or black olives

1. Mix oregano and vinaigrette dressing in a medium salad bowl. Add cucumber, green bell pepper, and olives. Toss with dressing and serve.

Preparation time: 10 minutes ● Servings: 2

Calories 77 ● Calories from Fat 28 ● Total Fat 3.2 g ● Saturated Fat 0.5 g ● Monounsaturated Fat 1.6 g ● Cholesterol 1 mg ● Sodium 150 mg ● Carbohydrate 11.5 g ● Dietary Fiber 4.0 g ● Sugars 5.9 g ● Protein 2.3 g

Exchanges: 2 vegetable, 1/2 fat

HELPFUL HINTS:

■ Roast chicken can be substituted for roast beef.

■ Diced fresh onions and tomatoes can be found in the produce section of the supermarket.

SHOPPING LIST

Deli
6 ounces sliced lean deli roast beef **/**

Grocery
1 package whole-wheat pita breads (6 1/2 inches each)
1 bottle dried oregano
1 bottle/can green or black olives

Produce
1 container fresh diced tomato
1 container fresh diced onion
1 bunch cilantro
1 cucumber
1 large green bell pepper

Staples
Balsamic vinegar
Reduced-fat vinaigrette dressing **/**
Salt
Black peppercorns

/ SHOP SMART!

Oven-roasted, no-salt-added, choice roast beef (per ounce): 45 calories, 1.7 g fat, 0.75 g saturated fat, 20 mg sodium
[*Example*: Boars Head brand]

Reduced-fat vinaigrette or oil and vinegar dressing (per tablespoon): 11 calories, 1.0 g fat, 4 mg sodium

SPAGHETTI BOLOGNESE (SPAGHETTI AND MEAT SAUCE) WITH HERBED ZUCCHINI

This simple, satisfying Italian meal features *spaghetti bolognese* with a side dish of herbed zucchini. The gastronomic city of Bologna claims to be the home of this famous dish. In this recipe, the addition of a little orange zest gives a sweet flavor to the sauce. If pressed for time, you can eliminate the vegetables and crushed tomatoes and use a bottled sauce instead. Add the orange zest to it.

Spaghetti Bolognese (Spaghetti and Meat Sauce)

1 teaspoon olive oil
1/2 cup fresh diced onions
1/2 cup fresh diced celery
1 teaspoon minced garlic
1/2 pound 95% lean ground beef

1/4 cup dry white wine
1 1/2 cups canned diced tomatoes ⚡
Zest from 1 orange (about 1/2 teaspoon)
Salt and freshly ground black pepper
1/4 pound whole-wheat spaghetti

COUNTDOWN

- Place water for pasta on to boil.
- Start Bolognese sauce.
- Make zucchini.
- Boil spaghetti.

1. Place a large pot with 3–4 quarts water on to boil over high heat.
2. Heat oil in a nonstick skillet over medium-high heat. Add onion and celery. Sauté 5 minutes, without browning. Add garlic and beef, crumbling the beef with a spoon as it cooks. Sauté 2 minutes.
3. Add white wine. Cook until the liquid is absorbed, about 1 minute.
4. Add the tomatoes and orange zest, and gently simmer, uncovered, for 15 minutes. Add salt and pepper to taste.
5. Meanwhile, add spaghetti to boiling water. Cook 9 minutes or according to package instructions. Drain pasta, and serve sauce over pasta.

Preparation time: 20 minutes ● Servings: 2

Calories 453 ● Calories from Fat 82 ● Total Fat 9.1 g ● Saturated Fat 3.1 g ● Monounsaturated Fat 4.2 g ● Cholesterol 144 mg ● Sodium 123 mg ● Carbohydrate 56.2 g ● Dietary Fiber 7.7 g ● Sugars 8.9 g ● Protein 34.9 g

Exchanges: 3 starch, 2 vegetable, 3 lean meat, 1/2 fat

Herbed Zucchini

2 medium zucchini, thinly sliced (2 cups)
1 teaspoon olive oil
1 teaspoon dried oregano
Salt and freshly ground black pepper

1. Place zucchini in a microwave-safe bowl. Cover and microwave on high 3 minutes. Or, bring water to a boil in a saucepan and add the zucchini. Cook 5 minutes. Drain, leaving about 2 tablespoons water in the pan. Return zucchini to the pot.
2. Toss the cooked zucchini with olive oil and oregano. Add salt and pepper to taste and serve.

Preparation time: 10 minutes ● Servings: 2

Calories 40 ● Calories from Fat 23 ● Total Fat 2.5 g ● Saturated Fat 0.5 g ● Monounsaturated Fat 1.7 g ● Cholesterol 0 mg ● Sodium 11 mg ● Carbohydrate 4.1 g ● Dietary Fiber 1.4 g ● Sugars 2.0 g ● Protein 1.4 g

Exchanges: 1 vegetable, 1/2 fat

HELPFUL HINTS:

■ Diced fresh onions and celery can be found in the produce section of the supermarket.

■ Slice zucchini in a food processor fitted with the thin slicing blade.

■ 95% lean ground beef is available in most supermarkets. Ask for it if you do not see it in the case.

SHOPPING LIST

Meat
1/2 pound 95% lean ground beef

Grocery
1 bottle or half bottle dry white wine
1 large can diced tomatoes **!**
1/4 pound whole-wheat spaghetti
1 bottle dried oregano

Produce
1 container fresh diced onions
1 container fresh diced celery
1 orange
2 medium zucchini

Staples
Olive oil
Minced garlic
Salt
Black peppercorns

! SHOP SMART!

Canned low-sodium diced tomatoes (per cup): 41 calories, 9.6 g carbohydrate, 24 mg sodium

STEAK AND PORTOBELLO SANDWICH WITH TAPENADE-TOPPED TOMATOES

Steak, mushrooms, and sweet onions are sautéed in the same pan to make this quick sandwich. The balsamic vinegar and garlic marinade becomes a dipping sauce for the sandwich. Meaty Portobello mushrooms are perfect for this dish. Buy whole ones, and slice them after they're cooked.

A tapenade is a thick paste made from capers, olives, oil, and vinegar. You can find it in jars in the grocery section.

Steak and Portobello Sandwich

3/4 pound grass-fed strip steak (3/4-inch thick)

2 teaspoons minced garlic

1/2 cup balsamic vinegar

1/4 pound whole Portobello mushrooms (1 2/3 cups when sliced)

4 slices whole-wheat bread (1 ounce each)

Olive oil spray

4 slices Vidalia onion

Salt and freshly ground black pepper

COUNTDOWN

■ Marinate steak.

■ While steak marinates, toast rolls and assemble tomatoes.

■ Finish sandwich.

1. Remove visible fat from steak.

2. Mix garlic and balsamic vinegar together in a self-sealing plastic bag. Add the steak and mushrooms. Marinate 10 minutes, turning bag over once during that time.

3. While the steak and mushrooms marinate, spray bread with olive oil spray. Toast in a toaster oven for 1 minute.

4. Heat a medium skillet over medium-high heat. Spray with olive oil spray. Remove steak and mushrooms from marinade, reserve marinade. Pat steak dry with a paper towel. Add steak to the skillet and sauté 3 minutes; turn and sauté 2–3 more minutes. A thermometer should read 145°F for medium-rare.

5. Transfer steak to a cutting board. Add the mushroom and onions to the skillet, and cook 5 minutes, turning over once. Transfer to the board with the steak. Sprinkle with salt and pepper to taste.

6. Add the reserved marinade to the skillet, and boil 3 minutes to reduce by half. Divide sauce between two small bowls to be used for dipping.

7. Slice steak and mushrooms into thin strips. Arrange meat and mushrooms on the bottom half of the bread. Place onions on top. Cover with the top slice of bread, and cut sandwich in half. Serve with the dipping sauce.

Preparation time: 30 minutes ● Servings: 2

Calories 438 ● Calories from Fat 74 ● Total Fat 8.2 g ● Saturated Fat 2.4 g ● Monounsaturated Fat 3.6 g ● Cholesterol 96 mg ● Sodium 385 mg ● Carbohydrate 41.0 g ● Dietary Fiber 5.1 g ● Sugars 14.0 g ● Protein 49.4 g

Exchanges: 2 starch, 1 vegetable, 6 lean meat

Tapenade-Topped Tomatoes

2 medium ripe tomatoes, sliced
2 tablespoons olive tapenade

1. Place tomatoes on a plate.
2. Spoon tapenade on top and serve.

Preparation time: 2 minutes ● Servings: 2

Calories 67 ● Calories from Fat 35 ● Total Fat 3.9 g ● Saturated Fat 0.6 g
● Monounsaturated Fat 0.1 g ● Cholesterol 0 mg ● Sodium 159 mg ●
Carbohydrate 8.1 g ● Dietary Fiber 2.2 g ● Sugars 4.7 g ● Protein 1.6 g

Exchanges: 1 vegetable, 1 fat

HELPFUL HINTS:

■ If grass-fed strip steak is unavailable, use 1/2 pound beef tenderloin.

■ Any type of whole-grain bread or roll can be used.

■ If Vidalia onions are not available, use another sweet onion, such as Texas 1015's or a red onion.

■ Minced garlic can be found in the produce section of the market.

SHOPPING LIST

Meat
3/4 lb grass-fed strip steak
   (3/4-inch thick)

Grocery
1 jar olive tapenade

Produce
1/4 pound whole Portobello
   mushrooms
1 Vidalia or other sweet onion
2 medium ripe tomatoes

Staples
Olive oil spray
Minced garlic
Balsamic vinegar
Whole-wheat bread
Salt
Black peppercorns

WALNUT-CRUSTED BUFFALO STEAK WITH TOMATO AND BEAN SALAD

Buffalo (or bison) is now available in most supermarkets, either fresh or frozen. It's a tasty alternative to beef and very low in saturated fat. With a walnut topping and a Tomato and Bean Salad, this meal is perfect for any occasion, whether ordinary or special. The nut coating provides a crunchy texture that contrasts with the tender meat. Hot pepper jelly gives this dish a surprising punch.

Walnut-Crusted Buffalo Steak

Olive oil spray
3/4 pound top sirloin buffalo steak
   (about 3/4-inch thick)

2 tablespoons hot pepper jam or jelly
2 tablespoons finely chopped walnuts
Salt and freshly ground black pepper

COUNTDOWN

■ Make salad and set aside.
■ Make steak.

1. Heat a nonstick skillet over medium-high heat. Spray with olive oil spray.
2. Add steak. Cook 3 minutes. Turn and spread the hot pepper jelly over the cooked side.
3. Press the walnuts into the steak. Continue to sauté the steak for 3 minutes for medium-rare. A meat thermometer should read 145°F. Sprinkle with salt and pepper to taste. Serve.

Preparation time: 10 minutes ● Servings: 2

Calories 308 ● Calories from Fat 92 ● Total Fat 10.3 g ● Saturated Fat 2.2 g ● Monounsaturated Fat 3.3 g ● Cholesterol 120 mg ● Sodium 91.4 mg ● Carbohydrate 14.6 g ● Dietary Fiber 0.6 g ● Sugars 8.0 g ● Protein 37.6 g

Exchanges: 1 carbohydrate, 5 lean meat

Tomato and Bean Salad

2 medium tomatoes, cut into large cubes (about 2 cups)
1 cup small Great Northern beans, drained and rinsed
2 tablespoons reduced-fat Italian salad (oil and vinegar, not creamy) dressing **!**
Salt and freshly ground black pepper
2 tablespoons chopped parsley (*optional*)

1. Place tomatoes and beans in a bowl. Add dressing. Toss well.

2. Add salt and pepper to taste, and mix again. Sprinkle parsley on top (if desired) and serve.

Preparation time: 5 minutes ● Servings: 2

Calories 194 ● Calories from Fat 17 ● Total Fat 1.9 g ● Saturated Fat 0.3 g ● Monounsaturated Fat 0.4 g ● Cholesterol 1 mg ● Sodium 20 mg ● Carbohydrate 35.5 g ● Dietary Fiber 8.7 g ● Sugars 5.4 g ● Protein 11.4 g

Exchanges: 2 starch, 1 vegetable

HELPFUL HINTS:

■ Chop the nuts in a food processor.

■ Any type of hot pepper jam or jelly can be used.

■ Any type of canned beans can be used for the salad.

■ Reduced-fat oil and vinegar dressing can be used instead of Italian dressing.

SHOPPING LIST

Meat
3/4 pound top sirloin buffalo steak

Grocery
1 jar hot pepper jam or jelly
1 small package walnuts
1 can small Great Northern beans
1 bottle reduced-fat Italian salad (oil and vinegar, not creamy) dressing **!**

Produce
2 medium tomatoes
1 bunch parsley (*optional*)

Staples
Olive oil spray
Salt
Black peppercorns

! SHOP SMART!

Reduced-fat Italian dressing—oil and vinegar, not creamy (per tablespoon): 11 calories, 1.0 g fat, 4 mg sodium

VIETNAMESE HOT AND SPICY STIR-FRY BEEF AND CHINESE NOODLES WITH SNOW PEAS

This dinner hosts a tasty blend of Pacific Rim flavors. Lemongrass is the secret flavor in this hot and spicy beef. It adds a tang like that of lemon or lime and is one of the most important spices in Thai cooking. It looks a little like a scallion with long, thin, green-gray leaves and a lighter bulb at the tip. Grated lemon rind can be used instead.

It will take several minutes to assemble and prepare the ingredients for this meal, but only a few minutes to cook them. This dinner is cooked in 5–7 minutes.

Vietnamese Hot and Spicy Stir-Fry Beef

1/4 cup tomato paste
1/2 teaspoon hot pepper sauce
1/2 cup water
2 teaspoons ground ginger
Olive oil spray
1/2 cup fresh diced onion
3 teaspoons minced garlic

1/2 cup sliced lemongrass, bulb end only, or grated lemon rind from 1 lemon
6 ounces beef tenderloin steak, cut into 1/2-inch by 2-inch strips
3 tablespoons broken walnuts
Salt and freshly ground black pepper

COUNTDOWN

■ Prepare ingredients.
■ Microwave noodles.
■ Stir-fry beef dish.
■ Stir-fry noodles.

1. Mix tomato paste, hot pepper sauce, water, and ginger together. Set aside.
2. Heat a wok or skillet over high heat, and spray with olive oil spray.
3. Add onion, garlic, and lemongrass (or lemon rind), and stir-fry 1 minute.
4. Add meat. Stir-fry 2 minutes.
5. Add sauce, and mix for a few seconds. Transfer to a plate, and sprinkle with walnuts, add salt and pepper to taste, and serve.

Preparation time: 5 minutes ● Servings: 2

Calories 292 ● Calories from Fat 131 ● Total Fat 14.6 g ● Saturated Fat 3.0 g ● Monounsaturated Fat 4.3 g ● Cholesterol 54 mg ● Sodium 120 mg ● Carbohydrate 20.0 g ● Dietary Fiber 3.2 g ● Sugars 6.1 g ● Protein 23.3 g

Exchanges: 4 vegetable, 2 lean meat, 2 fat

Chinese Noodles and Snow Peas

3 ounces Chinese noodles
2 cups frozen snow peas, thawed
1 teaspoon sesame oil
Salt and freshly ground black pepper

Microwave method

1. Place noodles in a microwave-safe bowl. Add 1/2 cup water. Cover and microwave on high 3 minutes. Add snow peas, sesame oil, and salt and pepper to taste. Transfer to two dinner plates, and serve meat on top.

Stove-top method

1. Bring a large saucepan filled with water to a boil. Add noodles; cook 1 minute. Add snow peas. Drain. Add salt and pepper to taste.

2. When meat is removed from wok, add sesame oil to wok and then the noodles and snow peas. Stir-fry 1 minute. Transfer to dinner plates, and serve beef on top.

Preparation time: 5 minutes ● Servings: 2

Calories 204 ● Calories from Fat 27 ● Total Fat 3.0 g ● Saturated Fat 0.5 g ● Monounsaturated Fat 1.0 g ● Cholesterol 0 mg ● Sodium 5 mg ● Carbohydrate 36.7 g ● Dietary Fiber 3.0 g ● Sugars 3.7 g ● Protein 7.3 g

Exchanges: 2 starch, 1 vegetable, 1/2 fat

HELPFUL HINTS:

■ Diced fresh onions can be found in the produce section of the supermarket.

■ Remove the woody outer leaves from the lemongrass before slicing. Cut pale inner leaves and the bulb into thin slices.

■ Prepare all ingredients for beef and noodle dishes before starting to stir-fry.

■ To save cleaning time, make stir-fry beef, transfer to a plate, and use the same wok for the noodles. You don't need to wash the wok between uses.

SHOPPING LIST

Beef
6 ounces beef tenderloin steak

Grocery
1/4 pound Chinese noodles
1 bottle sesame oil
1 small can tomato paste
1 bottle ground ginger
1 small package broken walnuts
1 package frozen snow peas

Produce
1 container fresh diced onion
3 stalks lemongrass or 1 lemon

Staples
Olive oil spray
Minced garlic
Hot pepper sauce
Salt
Black peppercorns

VEAL & LAMB

Veal and Olive Stew with Quick Barley	236
Quick-Fried Diced Veal with Simple Fried Rice	238
Scaloppini al Marsala (Veal Marsala) with Penne ala Siciliana (Sicilian Penne Pasta)	240
Veal Milanese with Spaghettini Pomodoro	242
Veau aux Oranges (Veal in Orange Sauce) and Broccoli Rice Pilaf	244
Lamb and Lentil Tagine	246
Middle-Eastern Lamb with Spinach Brown Rice	248

VEAL AND OLIVE STEW WITH QUICK BARLEY

A stew in just 20 minutes? It's true! In addition to being quick, you'll love this veal stew's rich, earthy flavors. It takes a few minutes to gather the ingredients for these recipes, but then they cook on their own.

Veal and Olive Stew

Olive oil spray
3/4 pound veal, cut from the leg into 1-inch cubes
1 cup fresh diced onion
2 teaspoons minced garlic
1/2 cup dry white wine

1 cup low-sodium canned crushed tomatoes
1/4 pound broccoli florets (about 1 1/2 cups)
8 black pitted olives, cut in half
1/2 cup fresh basil, torn into bite-size pieces (*optional*)
Salt and freshly ground black pepper

COUNTDOWN

■ Start veal.
■ While veal cooks, make barley.

1. Heat a nonstick skillet over medium-high heat, and spray with olive oil spray. Brown veal on all sides for 3 minutes.

2. Transfer veal to a plate. Add onion and garlic to skillet, and cook 1 minute. Add the wine, and cook 1 minute.

3. Add tomatoes and broccoli. Lower heat to medium-low, and return veal to the pan. Cover and simmer 10 minutes.

4. Add olives. Cook 5 minutes. Add basil (*optional*), salt and pepper to taste, and serve.

Preparation time: 20 minutes ● Servings: 2

Calories 346 ● Calories from Fat 73 ● Total Fat 8.1 g ● Saturated Fat 1.8 g ● Monounsaturated Fat 3.9 g ● Cholesterol 144 mg ● Sodium 333 mg ● Carbohydrate 20.4 g ● Dietary Fiber 3.3 g ● Sugars 6.9 g ● Protein 38.8 g

Exchanges: 4 vegetable, 5 lean meat, 1/2 fat

Quick Barley

1 1/2 cups water
1/2 cup quick-cooking pearl barley
2 teaspoons olive oil
Salt and freshly ground black pepper

1. Bring water to a boil in medium saucepan over high heat. Add barley. Reduce heat to medium, and simmer 10 minutes, covered.
2. Drain. Add oil, salt and pepper to taste, and serve.

Preparation time: 15 minutes ● Servings: 2

Calories 216 ● Calories from Fat 46 ● Total Fat 5.1 g ● Saturated Fat 0.7 g ● Monounsaturated Fat 3.4 g ● Cholesterol 0 mg ● Sodium 5 mg ● Carbohydrate 38.9 g ● Dietary Fiber 7.8 g ● Sugars 0.4 g ● Protein 5.0 g

Exchanges: 2 1/2 starch, 1/2 fat

HELPFUL HINT:

■ Look for quick-cooking barley in the supermarket.

■ Use veal cut from the leg. It will be tender. If this isn't available, ask the butcher for a quick-cooking cut of veal.

■ Diced fresh onions can be found in the produce section of the supermarket.

■ Minced garlic can be found in jars in the produce or condiment sections of the supermarket.

SHOPPING LIST

Meat
1/2 pound veal, cut from the leg into 1-inch cubes

Grocery
1 small bottle dry white wine
1 container black pitted olives
1 package quick-cooking pearl barley

Produce
1 container fresh diced/chopped onion
1 can low-sodium crushed tomatoes !
1/4 pound broccoli florets
1 bunch basil (*optional*)

Staples
Olive oil spray
Olive oil
Minced garlic
Salt
Black peppercorns

! SHOP SMART!

Canned crushed tomatoes (per cup): 41 calories, 0.3 g fat, 9.6 g carbohydrate, 24 mg sodium

QUICK-FRIED DICED VEAL WITH SIMPLE FRIED RICE

This stir-fried Chinese veal can be made faster than ordering takeout. It takes several minutes to gather the ingredients for stir-fry dishes, but only a few minutes to cook. Line up all of the ingredients on a plate or cutting board in the order that you will use them; then you won't have to keep referring to the recipe while cooking.

Sherry is combined with soy sauce to make a flavorful sauce. Fat-free low-sodium chicken broth can be used instead. The flavor will be different, but tasty.

Quick-Fried Diced Veal

1/2 cup sherry
1 1/2 tablespoons reduced-sodium soy sauce
4 teaspoons minced garlic
3/4 pound veal cutlet

1/2 tablespoon cornstarch
1/2 tablespoon sesame oil
2 cups peeled cucumber cubes

COUNTDOWN

- Marinate veal.
- Prepare other ingredients.
- Microwave rice.
- Stir-fry veal dish.
- Stir-fry rice.

1. In a small bowl, mix sherry, soy sauce, and garlic together. Cut veal into 1-inch pieces, and add to marinade. Set aside while preparing remaining ingredients.
2. Remove veal from marinade, reserving marinade. Toss veal in cornstarch, and set aside.
3. Heat sesame oil in a wok or skillet over high heat. Add veal, and stir-fry 1 minute. Add the marinade and cucumber. Stir-fry 2 minutes. Transfer to a plate. Use the same wok for the rice dish.

Preparation time: 10 minutes ● Servings: 2

Calories 323 ● Calories from Fat 61 ● Total Fat 6.8 g ● Saturated Fat 1.4 g ● Monounsaturated Fat 2.3 g ● Cholesterol 132 mg ● Sodium 518 mg ● Carbohydrate 14.8 g ● Dietary Fiber 1.3 g ● Sugars 2.0 g ● Protein 38.4 g

Exchanges: 1/2 carbohydrate, 1 vegetable, 5 lean meat, 1/2 alcohol

Simple Fried Rice

1 package microwaveable brown rice (to make 1 1/2 cups)
1/2 tablespoon sesame oil
1/2 cup frozen peas, thawed
Salt and freshly ground black pepper

1. Cook rice according to package instructions. Measure out 1 1/2 cups rice, and reserve remaining rice for another meal.
2. Heat sesame oil in the wok over high heat.
3. Add the rice and peas. Stir-fry 1 minute. Add salt and pepper to taste.
4. Divide between two dinner plates, and serve veal and sauce on top.

Preparation time: 5 minutes ● Servings: 2

Calories 238 ● Calories from Fat 55 ● Total Fat 6.1 g ● Saturated Fat 0.9 g ● Monounsaturated Fat 2.1 g ● Cholesterol 0 mg ● Sodium 52 mg ● Carbohydrate 34.2 g ● Dietary Fiber 3.0 g ● Sugars 1.9 g ● Protein 5.6 g

Exchanges: 2 1/2 starch, 1 fat

HELPFUL HINTS:

■ Boneless, skinless chicken breast can be substituted for the veal.

■ Minced garlic can be found in jars in the produce or condiment sections of the supermarket.

■ Your wok or skillet should be very hot, so the veal will be crisp.

■ If you're short on time, skip the rice recipe and serve the stir-fried veal over plain rice.

SHOPPING LIST

Meat
3/4 pound veal cutlet

Grocery
1 small bottle sherry
1 bottle reduced-sodium soy sauce
1 bottle sesame oil
1 package microwaveable brown rice
1 package frozen peas

Produce
1 cucumber

Staples
Minced garlic
Cornstarch
Salt
Black peppercorns

SCALOPPINI AL MARSALA (VEAL MARSALA) WITH PENNE ALA SICILIANA (SICILIAN PENNE PASTA)

Bring a touch of Sicily to your table with this succulent veal dressed in a sweet Marsala wine sauce, graced with a side of perfect pasta. Marsala wine is a sweet fortified wine that is produced by Sicilian families who have owned their vineyards for many generations.

Scaloppini al Marsala (Veal Marsala)

1 teaspoon olive oil
1/2 cup fresh diced onion
2 tablespoons flour
Salt and freshly ground black pepper

3/4 pound veal cutlets (about 1/2-inch thick)
1/3 cup Marsala wine
1/4 cup water

COUNTDOWN

- Place water for pasta on to boil.
- Make pasta dish.
- Make veal dish.

1. Heat the oil in a nonstick skillet over medium-high heat. Add the onion. Sauté without browning, about 2 minutes.
2. Place the flour on a plate, and add salt and pepper to taste. Dip the veal cutlets in the flour, making sure both sides are coated. Shake off excess flour.
3. Add veal to the onion in the skillet. Sauté 1 minute per side, and remove from the skillet. The veal should be almost cooked through.
4. Raise the heat to high. Add Marsala and water to the skillet. Reduce the liquid by half, about 1–2 minutes.
5. Remove skillet from the heat, return the veal to the skillet, and turn over in the sauce. Serve the veal on individual dinner plates, and spoon the sauce on top.

Preparation time: 10 minutes ● Servings: 2

Calories 304 ● Calories from Fat 48 ● Total Fat 5.4 g ● Saturated Fat 1.2 g ● Monounsaturated Fat 2.6 g ● Cholesterol 132 mg ● Sodium 113 mg ● Carbohydrate 14.4 g ● Dietary Fiber 0.9 g ● Sugars 4.8 g ● Protein 37.5 g

Exchanges: 1/2 carbohydrate, 1 vegetable, 5 lean meat

Penne ala Sicialianna (Sicilian Penne Pasta)

1/4 pound whole-wheat penne pasta (about 1 1/2 cups)
2 teaspoons olive oil
1 cup canned artichoke hearts, drained and cut in half
Salt and freshly ground black pepper
2 tablespoons chopped parsley (*optional*)

1. Place a large pot with 3–4 quarts water on to boil over high heat. Add the pasta to the water, and boil 10 minutes or according to package instructions.
2. Transfer 2 tablespoons cooking water to a bowl, and add olive oil.
3. Drain pasta. Add pasta and artichoke hearts to bowl. Add salt and pepper to taste. Toss well. Sprinkle parsley on top (if desired) and serve with veal.

Preparation time: 15 minutes ● Servings: 2

Calories 274 ● Calories from Fat 48 ● Total Fat 5.3 g ● Saturated Fat 0.8 g ● Monounsaturated Fat 3.4 g ● Cholesterol 0 mg ● Sodium 259 mg ● Carbohydrate 49.0 g ● Dietary Fiber 6.8 g ● Sugars 3.1 g ● Protein 10.5 g

Exchanges: 2 1/2 starch, 1 vegetable, 1/2 fat

SHOPPING LIST

Meat
3/4 pound veal cutlets (about 1/2-inch thick)

Grocery
1 small bottle Marsala wine
1 package whole-wheat penne pasta
1 can artichoke hearts

Produce
1 container fresh diced onion
1 bunch parsley (*optional*)

Staples
Olive oil
Flour
Salt
Black peppercorns

HELPFUL HINTS:

■ Sherry can be used instead of Marsala wine.

■ Boneless, skinless chicken breasts can be substituted for the veal. Flatten the breasts to about 1/2 inch, and cook them for about 3 minutes per side.

■ Any short-cut pasta can be used.

■ Diced fresh onions can be found in the produce section of the supermarket.

VEAL MILANESE WITH SPAGHETTINI POMODORO

Veal Milanese is a classic veal dish with a light, crisp breading. It is always a winner. Traditionally, this dish is served with pasta and tomato sauce.

The terms "cutlets" and "scallops" are both used when describing a cut of veal. In both cases, they refer to a thin cut that can be cooked quickly.

Veal Milanese

3/4 pound veal cutlets, about 1/2-inch thick
1/4 cup plain bread crumbs
2 tablespoons grated Parmesan cheese
Salt and freshly ground black pepper

1 egg white, slightly beaten
2 teaspoons olive oil
1 lemon, cut into wedges
1 tablespoon capers

COUNTDOWN

- Place water for pasta on to boil.
- Prepare veal ingredients.
- Add pasta to water.
- Make veal dish.
- Complete pasta dish.

1. Pound veal flat, to about 1/2 inch.
2. Mix bread crumbs and Parmesan cheese together, and add salt and pepper to taste.
3. Dip veal cutlets in egg white and then in a bread crumb mixture, making sure both sides are coated.
4. Heat oil in a nonstick skillet over medium-high heat, and add the cutlets. Cook 1 1/2 minutes; turn and cook second side 1 1/2 minutes. Divide between two dinner plates, and squeeze juice from lemon wedges on top.
5. Sprinkle with capers and salt and pepper to taste and serve.

Preparation time: 10 minutes ● Servings: 2

Calories 305 ● Calories from Fat 87 ● Total Fat 9.7 g ● Saturated Fat 2.6 g ● Monounsaturated Fat 4.8 g ● Cholesterol 136 mg ● Sodium 438 mg ● Carbohydrate 10.4 g ● Dietary Fiber 0.8 g ● Sugars 1.0 g ● Protein 41.8 g

Exchanges: 1 starch, 5 lean meat, 1 fat

Spaghettini Pomodoro

1/4 pound whole-wheat spaghettini
1 cup canned low-sodium diced tomatoes, drained ⚠
1/4 cup fresh basil leaves, torn into small pieces (*optional*)
Salt and freshly ground black pepper

1. Bring a large saucepan filled with water to a boil over high heat. Add the pasta, and cook 9–10 minutes or according to package instructions.
2. Drain. Toss pasta with diced tomatoes and fresh basil (if desired). Add salt and pepper to taste and serve.

Preparation time: 15 minutes ● Servings: 2

Calories 219 ● Calories from Fat 9 ● Total Fat 1.0 g ● Saturated Fat 0.2 g ● Monounsaturated Fat 0.1 g ● Cholesterol 0 mg ● Sodium 17 mg ● Carbohydrate 47.7 g ● Dietary Fiber 6.0 g ● Sugars 5.0 g ● Protein 9.4 g

Exchanges: 2 1/2 starch, 1 vegetable

HELPFUL HINTS:

■ Spaghettini is very thin spaghetti. Regular spaghetti can be used.

■ Thin-cut boneless, skinless chicken breasts can be used instead of veal. They should be about 1/2-inch thick.

SHOPPING LIST

Meat
3/4 pound veal cutlets, about 1/2-inch thick

Dairy
1 small piece Parmesan cheese

Grocery
1 container plain bread crumbs
1 bottle capers
1 package whole-wheat spaghettini
1 small can low-sodium diced tomatoes ⚠

Produce
1 lemon
1 bunch basil (*optional*)

Staples
Olive oil
Egg
Salt
Black peppercorns

⚠ **SHOP SMART!**

Canned low-sodium diced tomatoes (per cup): 41 calories, 9.6 g carbohydrate, 24 mg sodium

VEAU AUX ORANGES (VEAL IN ORANGE SAUCE) AND BROCCOLI RICE PILAF

Veal doesn't have to be a company-only dish. This dinner of Veal in Orange Sauce and Broccoli Rice Pilaf doesn't take long to make. In fact, the veal itself cooks in less than 5 minutes. The secret is to carefully cook the thin slices of veal. If veal is overcooked, it will be tough and dry and even a good sauce won't help.

A pilaf is a rice dish that originated in the Middle East. The rice is first sautéed in a skillet and then the liquid is added. For this dish, I added broccoli, but any type of vegetable can be used. Try zucchini or a mixture of vegetables, if you like.

Veau aux Oranges (Veal in Orange Sauce)

1/2 pound veal cutlets
1 teaspoon olive oil
Salt and freshly ground black pepper
3 medium shallots, chopped (1/4 cup)
1/4 cup sherry wine vinegar

1 teaspoon dried rosemary
1 teaspoon dried thyme
1/2 cup orange juice plus 2 tablespoons
2 teaspoons cornstarch

COUNTDOWN

■ Start rice.
■ While rice cooks, make veal.
■ When rice is finished, set aside, covered, and complete veal dish.

1. Remove visible fat from veal, and pound flat with the palm of your hand or the bottom of a heavy skillet to 1/4–1/2 inch.
2. Heat oil in a medium nonstick skillet over high heat. Brown veal on both sides, about 1 minute per side for veal that is 1/4-inch thick, 30 seconds longer for a thicker piece. Transfer to a plate. Sprinkle with salt and pepper to taste.
3. Add shallots and sherry wine vinegar to skillet. Sauté, scraping up brown bits in pan, until vinegar evaporates, about 1 minute.
4. Add rosemary, thyme, and 1/2 cup orange juice to pan. Simmer 1 minute.
5. Mix cornstarch and remaining 2 tablespoons orange juice together. Add to sauce. Simmer until sauce thickens, several seconds. Serve veal with sauce spooned over top.

Preparation time: 10 minutes ● Servings: 2

Calories 205 ● Calories from Fat 43 ● Total Fat 4.8 g ● Saturated Fat 1.1 g ● Monounsaturated Fat 2.4 g ● Cholesterol 88 mg ● Sodium 75 mg ● Carbohydrate 13.5 g ● Dietary Fiber 1.1 g ● Sugars 0 g ● Protein 25.2 g

Exchanges: 1 carbohydrate, 3 lean meat

Broccoli Rice Pilaf

1/2 pound broccoli florets cut into small pieces (about 3 cups)
Olive oil spray
1 teaspoon minced garlic
1/2 cup long-grain white rice
1 cup fat-free low-sodium chicken broth
Salt and freshly ground black pepper

1. Cut broccoli florets into 1/2-inch pieces. Heat a nonstick skillet over medium-high heat, and spray with olive oil spray. Add broccoli and garlic. Sauté 1 minute.

2. Add rice, and sauté 1 minute.

3. Add broth. Bring to a boil, cover, lower heat, and simmer, gently, 15 minutes. Rice should be cooked through and liquid absorbed. If rice seems a little dry, add a few tablespoons chicken broth. Add salt and pepper to taste and serve.

Preparation time: 20 minutes ● Servings: 2

Calories 226 ● Calories from Fat 19 ● Total Fat 2.2 g ● Saturated Fat 0.4 g ● Monounsaturated Fat 1.1 g ● Cholesterol 0 mg ● Sodium 321 mg ● Carbohydrate 44.8 g ● Dietary Fiber 0.7 g ● Sugars 0.1 g ● Protein 8.4 g

Exchanges: 2 1/2 starch, 1 vegetable

HELPFUL HINTS:

■ Boneless, skinless chicken can be used instead of veal. Cook 2 minutes per side for 1/4-inch-thick piece.

■ Balsamic vinegar can be used instead of sherry wine vinegar.

■ Minced garlic can be found in jars in the produce or condiment sections of the supermarket.

■ Sweet onions can be used instead of shallots.

■ Make sure your skillet is very hot before browning the veal. The juices will be sealed in and a brown crust will form.

SHOPPING LIST

Meat
1/2 pound veal cutlets

Grocery
1 bottle sherry wine vinegar
1 bottle dried rosemary
1 bottle dried thyme
1 small bottle orange juice

Produce
3 medium shallots
1/2 pound broccoli florets

Staples
Olive oil
Olive oil spray
Minced garlic
Long-grain white rice
Cornstarch
Fat-free low-sodium chicken broth
Salt
Black peppercorns

LAMB AND LENTIL TAGINE

Lamb cubes blend with fragrant spices in this pleasant Moroccan tagine. Tagines are cooked in a glazed earthenware dish with a conical lid. It's used for slow cooking the ingredients. Steam gathers in the top of the conical lid and falls on the food, keeping it moist without basting. However, any type of skillet or casserole can be used for this dinner. I've shortened the cooking time by using a skillet and using tender lamb that has been cut for lamb kabobs.

Lamb and Lentil Tagine

1 tablespoon olive oil

1/2 pound lamb cubes (cut from the leg or for kabobs), about 1-inch cubes

2 cups frozen chopped/diced onion

2 teaspoons minced garlic

2 medium tomatoes, cut into 8 wedges (about 2 cups)

1 teaspoon ground cinnamon

2 teaspoons ground cumin

Salt and freshly ground black pepper

2 cups water

1/2 cup dried lentils

6 cups washed ready-to-eat spinach

COUNTDOWN

■ Prepare ingredients.
■ Make tagine.

1. Heat oil in a medium nonstick skillet over high heat. Add the lamb cubes, and brown for 2 minutes, turning the cubes to make sure all sides are browned. Transfer lamb to a plate.

2. Add onion, garlic, tomato, cinnamon, cumin, and salt and black pepper to taste to skillet. Cook 1 minute to release the juices in the dried spices.

3. Add water and lentils. Bring the water to a simmer, reduce heat to medium, and gently simmer 20 minutes. The water should be absorbed. Stir in the lamb and spinach, and cook 2 minutes. Serve on two dinner plates.

Preparation time: 30 minutes ● Servings: 2

Calories 517 ● Calories from Fat 132 ● Total Fat 14.7 g ● Saturated Fat 3.4 g ● Monounsaturated Fat 7.8 g ● Cholesterol 74 mg ● Sodium 170 mg ● Carbohydrate 58.1 g ● Dietary Fiber 22.8 g ● Sugars 13.0 g ● Protein 42.0g

Exchanges: 2 starch, 3 vegetable, 5 lean meat, 1 fat

HELPFUL HINTS:

■ If lamb cut from the leg isn't available, ask the butcher for a quick-cooking cut of lamb.

■ Minced garlic can be found in jars in the produce or condiment sections of the supermarket.

■ If the skillet becomes dry before the lentils are cooked, add a little more water.

SHOPPING LIST

Meat
1/2 pound lamb cubes
   (cut from the leg)

Grocery
1 bottle ground cinnamon
1 bottle ground cumin
1 package dried lentils
1 package frozen chopped/diced
   onion

Produce
2 medium tomatoes
1 bag washed ready-to-eat spinach

Staples
Olive oil
Minced garlic
Salt
Black peppercorns

MIDDLE-EASTERN LAMB WITH SPINACH BROWN RICE

Eat quick with this delightful lamb dish featuring a Middle-Eastern sauce of garlic, ground cumin, cucumber, and yogurt. Look for lamb cut from the leg or for kabobs.

Middle-Eastern Lamb

1/2 cup nonfat plain yogurt
1 teaspoon minced garlic
1 teaspoon ground cumin
1/4 cup peeled, diced cucumber

Olive oil spray
1/2 pound lamb cubes, cut from the leg
Salt and freshly ground black pepper

COUNTDOWN

■ Prepare lamb sauce.
■ Make lamb.
■ Make rice.

1. Mix yogurt, garlic, cumin, and cucumber together. Set aside.

2. Heat a nonstick skillet over medium-high heat. Spray with olive oil spray.

3. Cut lamb into 1/2-inch pieces, and add to the skillet. Sauté 2 minutes, turning to brown on all sides. Sprinkle with salt and pepper to taste.

4. Transfer lamb to two dinner plates, spoon sauce on top, and serve.

Preparation time: 10 minutes ● Servings: 2

Calories 210 ● Calories from Fat 70 ● Total Fat 7.8 g ● Saturated Fat 2.4 g ● Monounsaturated Fat 3.6 g ● Cholesterol 75 mg ● Sodium 126 mg ● Carbohydrate 6.9 g ● Dietary Fiber 0.3 g ● Sugars 0.2 g ● Protein 26.9 g

Exchanges: 1/2 carbohydrate, 4 lean meat

Spinach Brown Rice

1 package microwaveable brown rice (for 1 1/2 cups rice)
5 cups washed ready-to-eat spinach
2 teaspoons olive oil
Salt and freshly ground black pepper

1. Microwave rice according to package instructions. Measure 1 1/2 cups cooked rice into a bowl. Reserve remaining rice for another meal.

2. Add spinach to warm rice, and toss well.

3. Add olive oil and salt and pepper to taste. Toss again and serve.

Preparation time: 5 minutes ● Servings: 2

Calories 238 ● Calories from Fat 66 ● Total Fat 7.3 g ● Saturated Fat 1.0 g ● Monounsaturated Fat 4.0 g ● Cholesterol 0 mg ● Sodium 71 mg ● Carbohydrate 32.0 g ● Dietary Fiber 3.3 g ● Sugars 0.3 g ● Protein 5.9 g

Exchanges: 2 starch, 1 vegetable, 1 fat

HELPFUL HINTS:

■ Minced garlic can be found in jars in the produce or condiment sections of the supermarket.

■ If lamb cut from the leg isn't available, ask the butcher for a quick-cooking cut of lamb.

SHOPPING LIST

Meat
6 ounces lamb cubes,
   cut from the leg

Grocery
1 carton nonfat plain yogurt
1 bottle ground cumin
1 package microwaveable brown rice

Produce
1 small cucumber
1 bag washed ready-to-eat spinach

Staples
Olive oil
Olive oil spray
Minced garlic
Salt
Black peppercorns

VEGETARIAN

Frittata Primavera with Gratinéed Fennel   252
Greek-Style Casserole Soup   254
Indian-Spiced Spinach with Lentils and Rice   256
Mulligatawny Soup   258
Ricotta Soufflé with Tomato Bruschetta   260
Southwestern Three-Bean Soup   262
Tabbouleh with Toasted Walnut Couscous   264
Mushroom Pesto Pasta with Pimento Salad   266

FRITTATA PRIMAVERA WITH GRATINÉED FENNEL

This is a light, quick supper, perfect for a busy weekday meal. Frittata Primavera is an Italian omelet filled with fresh vegetables. Cook it slowly for 10 minutes so that it becomes thick, more like a quiche than an omelet. Use fresh basil and good-quality fresh Parmesan cheese for the best results.

Fennel is sometimes called anise. It has a pale green bulb with feather-like leaves, similar to dill. It has a slightly sweet, licorice flavor when raw and a pleasant, very mild flavor when cooked.

Frittata Primavera

1/2 pound red potatoes (1 1/2 cups cubed)
1 tablespoon olive oil
1 cup fresh sliced onion
1 cup sliced baby bello mushrooms
1/2 cup fresh diced green bell pepper
1 teaspoon minced garlic
1/2 cup shelled fresh or frozen edamame

1 large whole egg
4 large egg whites
1/4 cup nonfat milk
1/2 cup fresh basil
Salt and freshly ground black pepper
2 slices whole-grain bread (1 ounce each)
Olive oil spray

COUNTDOWN

■ Preheat broiler.
■ Start potatoes.
■ While potatoes cook, prepare vegetables.
■ While frittata cooks, make fennel.
■ Complete frittata.

1. Preheat broiler.
2. Wash potatoes, do not remove skin, and cut into small cubes, about 1/4 inch.
3. Heat oil in a medium nonstick skillet over medium-high heat. Add potatoes, making sure they are in one layer, and sauté, tossing to brown all sides, 5 minutes.
4. While potatoes cook, measure onion, mushrooms, green pepper, and garlic. Add to skillet with the edamame, and continue to sauté 5 minutes.
5. Whisk whole egg, egg whites, and milk together. Tear basil into small pieces, and add to egg mixture with a little salt and pepper to taste. Pour into skillet. Gently stir vegetables to make sure egg mixture spreads throughout the pan.
6. Turn heat to low, and cook 10 minutes. Frittata will be mostly cooked through.
7. Place frittata under broiler to brown, 1–2 minutes. Watch to make sure top doesn't brown too much.
8. While frittata is in broiler, spray bread with olive oil spray and place bread in broiler under frittata pan or in oven to warm.
9. To serve, loosen frittata around edges, cut in half, and slip each half onto individual plates. Serve with warm bread.

Preparation time: 25 minutes ● Servings: 2

Calories 382 ● Calories from Fat 121 ● Total Fat 13.5 g ● Saturated Fat 1.9 g ● Monounsaturated Fat 6.5 g ● Cholesterol 107 mg ● Sodium 287 mg ● Carbohydrate 45.1g ● Dietary Fiber 7.5 g ● Sugars 7.6 g ● Protein 23.0 g

Exchanges: 2 1/2 starch, 1 vegetable, 2 lean meat, 1 1/2 fat

Gratinéed Fennel

1 fennel bulb, sliced (4 cups)
1/4 cup plain bread crumbs
3 tablespoons freshly grated Parmesan cheese

1. Remove feathery top of fennel and any outer leaves of the bulb that look damaged. Discard. Wash and slice bulb.

2. Spread slices over the bottom of a microwave-safe baking dish (about 8 by 10 inches).

3. Cover and microwave on high 5 minutes.

4. Mix bread crumbs and Parmesan cheese together. Sprinkle evenly over fennel. Place under broiler when frittata has been removed. Broil 1 minute. Remove from broiler and serve.

Preparation time: 10 minutes ● Servings: 2

Calories 140 ● Calories from Fat 29 ● Total Fat 3.2 g ● Saturated Fat 1.5 g ● Monounsaturated Fat 0.8 g ● Cholesterol 6 mg ● Sodium 303 mg ● Carbohydrate 22.7 g ● Dietary Fiber 6.0 g ● Sugars 0.9 g ● Protein 6.8 g

Exchanges: 1/2 starch, 2 vegetable, 1 fat

HELPFUL HINTS:

■ Sliced fresh onions and diced green bell pepper can be found in the produce section of the supermarket.

■ Use a nonstick skillet with an ovenproof handle for the frittata.

■ Slice the fennel in a food processor fitted with a slicing blade.

■ Use a baking dish that fits in a microwave oven for the fennel.

■ If a microwave is not available, place fennel in a large saucepan of boiling water. Boil 5 minutes and drain. Place in an ovenproof dish and continue with recipe.

SHOPPING LIST

Dairy
1 small package Parmesan cheese
Nonfat milk

Grocery
1 package shelled fresh or frozen edamame
1 loaf whole-grain bread

Produce
1/2 pound red potatoes
1 package fresh sliced onion
1 package sliced baby bello mushrooms
1 package fresh diced green bell pepper
1 bunch basil
1 fennel bulb

Staples
Olive oil
Olive oil spray
Minced garlic
Plain bread crumbs
Eggs (5 needed)
Salt
Black peppercorns

GREEK-STYLE CASSEROLE SOUP

Vegetables and Arborio rice dress up this hearty soup, which takes only 20 minutes to make. It's a whole meal in a single bowl. My family, no matter what the weather, loves a bowl of soup; but usually, soups take too long to make for a midweek meal. This quick meal fits the bill.

Arborio rice is an Italian rice that is shorter and plumper than other short-grained rice varieties. It's used to make creamy Italian risotto.

Greek-Style Casserole Soup

1 tablespoon olive oil

1 cup frozen chopped or diced onion

1/2 pound sliced zucchini (about 2 cups)

1 cup fresh diced celery

1 teaspoon minced garlic

1 cup organic vegetable broth ⚡

1 cup canned low-sodium whole tomatoes, drained ⚡

1 cup water

1/3 cup Arborio rice, uncooked

4 cups washed ready-to-eat spinach

1/2 teaspoon dried thyme

Salt and freshly ground black pepper

2 tablespoons crumbled feta cheese

1/4 cup unsalted pistachios

COUNTDOWN

■ Prepare ingredients.

■ Make soup.

1. Heat oil in a large saucepan over medium-high heat. Add onion, zucchini, celery, and garlic. Sauté 2–3 minutes.

2. Add the broth, tomatoes, water, and rice. Break up the tomatoes with the edge of a spoon. Bring soup to a simmer, cover, and cook 15 minutes.

3. Add spinach and thyme. Cook until the spinach is wilted, about 1 minute. Add salt and pepper to taste.

4. Spoon into two soup bowls, and sprinkle feta cheese, nuts, and salt and pepper to taste on top. Serve.

Preparation time: 25 minutes ● Servings: 2

Calories 390 ● Calories from Fat 150 ● Total Fat 16.7 g ● Saturated Fat 3.4 g ● Monounsaturated Fat 9.1 g ● Cholesterol 8 mg ● Sodium 498 mg ● Carbohydrate 52.5 g ● Dietary Fiber 8.1 g ● Sugars 8.8 g ● Protein 12.4 g

Exchanges: 2 1/2 starch, 3 vegetable, 3 fat

HELPFUL HINTS:

■ Use a medium- or short-grained rice if Arborio rice is unavailable.

■ Domestic crumbled feta cheese is available in most markets and works well for this recipe.

■ Diced fresh celery can be found in the produce section of the supermarket.

SHOPPING LIST

Dairy
1 small package crumbled feta cheese

Grocery
1 package frozen chopped or diced onion
1 can organic vegetable broth **!**
1 can low-sodium whole tomatoes **!**
1 package Arborio rice
1 bottle dried thyme
1 package shelled unsalted pistachios

Produce
1/2 pound sliced zucchini
1 container fresh diced celery
1 bag washed ready-to-eat spinach

Staples
Olive oil
Minced garlic
Salt
Black peppercorns

! SHOP SMART!

Organic vegetable broth (per cup): 12 calories, 3.0 g carbohydrate, 550 mg sodium

Low-sodium canned whole tomatoes (per cup): 41 calories, 0.3 g fat, 9.6 g carbohydrate, 24 mg sodium

INDIAN-SPICED SPINACH WITH LENTILS AND RICE

Cumin and coriander add a taste of India to this spinach dish. Onion, pine nuts, and garlic complete the exciting exotic flavor. The Lentils and Rice takes less than 5 minutes to make if you are using microwaveable brown rice.

Indian-Spiced Spinach

Olive oil spray
1 cup fresh diced onion
2 teaspoons minced garlic
2 cups canned low-sodium diced tomatoes, drained 🔳
8 cups washed ready-to-eat spinach
2 teaspoons ground cumin

2 teaspoons ground coriander
1/8 teaspoon cayenne pepper
1/4 cup pine nuts
2 teaspoons olive oil
Salt and freshly ground black pepper

COUNTDOWN

■ Start spinach.
■ While spinach cooks, make rice.
■ Finish spinach.
■ Complete rice dish.

1. Heat a large nonstick skillet over medium-high heat, and spray with olive oil spray.
2. Add onion and garlic. Sauté 3 minutes, stirring to prevent burning.
3. Add tomatoes and spinach, cover, and cook 5 minutes.
4. Remove lid, and add cumin, coriander, cayenne, and pine nuts. Cook 5 minutes, uncovered. Stir in olive oil and salt and pepper to taste. Serve.

Preparation time: 15 minutes ● Servings: 2

Calories 258 ● Calories from Fat 141 ● Total Fat 15.7 g ● Saturated Fat 2.3 g ● Monounsaturated Fat 7.7 g ● Cholesterol 0 mg ● Sodium 131 mg ● Carbohydrate 26.0 g ● Dietary Fiber 8.2 g ● Sugars 8.7 g ● Protein 11.1 g

Exchanges: 4 vegetable, 3 fat

Lentils and Rice

1 package microwaveable brown rice (1 cup cooked rice)
1/2 cup canned lentils, rinsed and drained ⚠
1 tablespoon olive oil
Salt and freshly ground black pepper

1. Microwave rice according to package instructions. Measure 1 cup into a bowl, and reserve remaining rice for another meal.

2. Add lentils to rice.

3. Add oil and salt and pepper to taste. Toss well and serve.

Preparation time: 5 minutes ● Servings: 2

Calories 240 ● Calories from Fat 78 ● Total Fat 8.7g ● Saturated Fat 1.2 g ● Monounsaturated Fat 5.5 g ● Cholesterol 0 mg ● Sodium 110 mg ● Carbohydrate 30.0 g ● Dietary Fiber 3.5 g ● Sugars 0.5 g ● Protein 6.5 g

Exchanges: 2 starch, 1 1/2 fat

HELPFUL HINTS:

■ Spices lose their flavor and strength if kept too long. Make sure your cumin and coriander are no more than 6 months old.

■ Diced fresh onions can be found in the produce section of the supermarket.

SHOPPING LIST

Grocery
1 small can low-sodium diced tomatoes ⚠
1 bottle ground cumin
1 bottle ground coriander
1 small bottle cayenne pepper
1 package pine nuts
1 package microwaveable brown rice
1 can lentils ⚠

Produce
1 container fresh diced onion
1 bag washed ready-to-eat spinach

Staples
Olive oil
Olive oil spray
Minced garlic
Salt
Black peppercorns

⚠ SHOP SMART!

Canned low-sodium diced tomatoes (per cup): 41 calories, 9.6 g carbohydrate, 24 mg sodium

Canned lentils (per cup): 240 calories, 680 mg sodium

MULLIGATAWNY SOUP

Mulligatawny soup has Anglo-Indian origins. It's attributed to servants for the English Raj in India. Curry powder and ginger give the soup a pungent flavor, while freshly diced crunchy apple provide a contrast in texture. This soup tastes great the second day. If you have time, make double.

Authentic curry powder is a blend of freshly ground spices and herbs, such as cardamom, chilies, cinnamon, cloves, coriander, and cumin, and in authentic Indian homes and restaurants, it is made fresh every day. Commercial curry powder comes in two forms: standard and Madras, the hotter one.

Mulligatawny Soup

2 teaspoons canola oil
1 cup fresh sliced onion
1/2 cup sliced carrot
1/2 cup fresh diced celery
1/2 tablespoon curry powder
1 tablespoon flour
1 teaspoon ground ginger
1 1/2 cups fat-free, low-sodium organic vegetable broth

1 cup water
1/2 cup light coconut milk
1/2 cup dried lentils
Salt and freshly ground black pepper
1 cup cored and cubed apple
1/4 cup slivered almonds, toasted
2 tablespoons chopped fresh cilantro
2 lemon wedges

COUNTDOWN

■ Start soup.
■ While soup simmers, cut apple and toast almonds.
■ Complete soup.

1. Heat oil in a large saucepan over medium-high heat.
2. Add onion, carrot, and celery. Sauté 5 minutes, stirring occasionally. Add the curry powder, flour, and ginger, and sauté about 30 seconds.
3. Stir in vegetable broth, water, and coconut milk. Bring to a boil, and add lentils. Reduce heat to a simmer, and cover with a lid. Cook 20 minutes.
4. Add salt and pepper to taste. To serve, ladle soup into two bowls and sprinkle with cubed apple, almonds, and cilantro. Place lemon wedges on side.

Preparation time: 30 minutes ● Servings: 2

Calories 450 ● Calories from Fat 163 ● Total Fat 18.1 g ● Saturated Fat 3.1 g ● Monounsaturated Fat 8.9 g ● Cholesterol 0 mg ● Sodium 480 mg ● Carbohydrate 59.0 g ● Dietary Fiber 20.9 g ● Sugars 14.3 g ● Protein 19.0 g

Exchanges: 2 starch, 1/2 fruit, 2 vegetable, 1 lean meat, 3 1/2 fat

HELPFUL HINTS:

■ Curry powder can be found in the spice section of the supermarket. It loses its freshness after 2–3 months.

■ Sliced fresh onions and diced fresh celery can be found in the produce section of the supermarket.

RICOTTA SOUFFLÉ WITH TOMATO BRUSCHETTA

This unusual soufflé tempts you with sautéed vegetables mixed with ricotta cheese and a topping of bread crumbs. It only takes 20 minutes to make. Spreading the mixture in a thin layer in a baking dish cuts down the cooking time. The zucchini and carrots are chopped and the mushrooms and onions are sliced to give a variety of textures. Using your food processor, you can prepare all of the vegetables in 5 minutes. Use the chopping blade first for the zucchini and carrots. Transfer vegetables to a bowl. Add the basil and chop. Transfer to another bowl.

Ricotta Soufflé

1 cup chopped zucchini
1 cup chopped carrots
2 1/2 cups sliced button mushrooms
1/2 cup fresh diced onion
2 teaspoons olive oil

3/4 cup chopped fresh basil, divided
1/2 cup plain bread crumbs
Salt and freshly ground black pepper
1 cup nonfat ricotta cheese
2 whole eggs

COUNTDOWN

- Preheat oven to 400°F.
- Make Ricotta Soufflé.
- Prepare bruschetta topping.
- Toast bread in a toaster oven or under the broiler.

1. Preheat oven to 400°F.
2. Add zucchini, carrots, mushrooms, and onion to an ovenproof dish or lasagna dish about 8 by 10 inches. Drizzle oil over vegetables. Cover and microwave on high 3 minutes.
3. Meanwhile, in a small bowl, mix 1/2 cup basil with bread crumbs, and add salt and pepper to taste.
4. Remove vegetables from microwave. Mix the ricotta cheese and eggs together, and add to the vegetables. Spread the vegetables evenly throughout the dish. Sprinkle bread crumb mixture on top. Bake 15 minutes.
5. Sprinkle remaining 1/4 cup chopped basil over the top and serve.

Preparation time: 25 minutes ● Servings: 2

Calories 377 ● Calories from Fat 104 ● Total Fat 11.5 g ● Saturated Fat 2.6 g ● Monounsaturated Fat 5.5 g ● Cholesterol 262 mg ● Sodium 478 mg ● Carbohydrate 39.8 g ● Dietary Fiber 11.1 g ● Sugars 7.4 g ● Protein 30.5 g

Exchanges: 1 starch, 4 vegetable, 3 lean meat, 1 fat

Tomato Bruschetta

1/4 whole-wheat baguette (2 slices)
1 medium clove garlic
1/4 cup cherry or grape tomatoes, cut in half and coarsely chopped
2 teaspoons olive oil
Salt and freshly ground black pepper

1. Line a baking tray with foil. Place bread on tray, and toast in toaster oven or under a broiler until golden, 3–4 minutes. Remove from oven.

2. Cut garlic in half. Rub cut halves over bread.

3. Toss tomato and olive oil together. Spoon over bread. Pour any excess oil left from mixing with tomatoes over bread.

4. Sprinkle with salt and pepper to taste and serve.

Preparation time: 10 minutes ● Servings: 2

Calories 121 ● Calories from Fat 48 ● Total Fat 5.3 g ● Saturated Fat 0.8 g ● Monounsaturated Fat 3.6 g ● Cholesterol 0 mg ● Sodium 137 mg ● Carbohydrate 15.9 g ● Dietary Fiber 1.3 g ● Sugars 0.6 g ● Protein 2.8 g

Exchanges: 1 starch, 1 fat

SHOPPING LIST

Dairy
1 small carton nonfat ricotta cheese

Grocery
1 whole-wheat baguette

Produce
1 zucchini
1 carrot
1 package sliced button mushrooms
1 package fresh diced onion
1 bunch basil
1 container cherry or grape tomatoes

Staples
Olive oil
Garlic
Eggs
Plain bread crumbs
Salt
Black peppercorns

HELPFUL HINTS

■ Any variety of vegetables can be substituted in this recipe. Simply make sure they are cooked through before adding the cheese.

■ Diced fresh onions can be found in the produce section of the supermarket.

■ Chop zucchini and carrots in a food processor.

■ If the ovenproof dish doesn't fit in your microwave, cook the vegetables in a bowl and transfer them to the ovenproof dish.

SOUTHWESTERN THREE-BEAN SOUP

This thick hearty soup is a great 25-minute supper. It also freezes well. If you have time, make double and have another meal ready for emergencies.

Southwestern Three-Bean Soup

2 1/4 cups water, divided
1 cup fresh sliced onion
1 cup shelled edamame
1/2 cup sliced parsnip
1/2 cup canned low-sodium red kidney beans, rinsed and drained
1/2 cup canned low-sodium chickpeas, rinsed and drained

1/2 cup frozen baby lima beans
1 cup canned low-sodium whole tomatoes with juice
2 teaspoons smoked paprika
2 teaspoons chili powder
1 tablespoon olive oil
Salt and freshly ground black pepper
2 tablespoons chopped fresh cilantro
1/4 cup reduced-fat shredded Mexican-style cheese

COUNTDOWN

■ Assemble ingredients.
■ Make soup.

1. Place a large saucepan over medium heat. Add 1/2 cup water, onion, edamame, and parsnip. Sauté 5 minutes.

2. Add kidney beans, chickpeas, lima beans, tomatoes, remaining 1 3/4 cups water, paprika, and chili powder. Break up tomatoes with a spoon or knife, and bring to a simmer. Simmer 20 minutes.

3. Stir in the olive oil. Add salt and pepper to taste. Serve in two bowls, and sprinkle with cilantro and cheese.

Preparation time: 30 minutes ● Servings: 2

Calories 441 ● Calories from Fat 127 ● Total Fat 14.1 g ● Saturated Fat 2.9 g ● Monounsaturated Fat 5.9 g ● Cholesterol 9 mg ● Sodium 283 mg ● Carbohydrate 60.6 g ● Dietary Fiber 15.3 g ● Sugars 5.7 g ● Protein 23.7 g

Exchanges: 3 starch, 2 vegetable, 2 lean meat, 1 1/2 fat

HELPFUL HINTS:

■ Fresh or frozen shelled edamame can be used.

■ A good-quality paprika can be substituted for smoked paprika.

■ Diced fresh onions can be found in the produce section of the supermarket.

TABBOULEH WITH TOASTED WALNUT COUSCOUS

Fresh mint, parsley, olive oil, and lemon juice brighten this Middle-Eastern dish. Bulgur wheat adds an earthy flavor and is made from wheat kernels that have been steamed, dried, and crushed. One secret to flavorful tabbouleh is to crush the scallions and wheat together, so the juices from the scallions penetrate the wheat.

Tabbouleh

1/2 cup uncooked fine bulgur wheat
4 scallions, sliced (about 3/4 cup)
1/2 cup chopped fresh flat leaf parsley
1/2 cup chopped fresh mint
1 tablespoon olive oil

2 tablespoons lemon juice
Salt and freshly ground black pepper
1 ripe medium tomato, cut into eighths (about 1 cup)
2 tablespoons sliced black olives

COUNTDOWN

- Soak bulgur wheat.
- Prepare ingredients.
- Start couscous.
- Complete tabbouleh.

1. Place bulgur wheat in a small bowl, and add cold water to cover. Let stand 20 minutes, while you prepare the other ingredients.
2. Drain and squeeze out as much water as possible from the wheat.
3. Add the scallions. Squeeze again with your hands, so the scallion juices penetrate the wheat.
4. Add parsley, mint, olive oil, and lemon juice. Toss well.
5. Add salt and pepper to taste.
6. Spoon onto individual plates, place tomatoes and olives on top, and serve.

Preparation time: 25 minutes ● Servings: 2

Calories 244 ● Calories from Fat 75 ● Total Fat 8.3 g ● Saturated Fat 1.2 g ● Monounsaturated Fat 5.6 g ● Cholesterol 0 mg ● Sodium 79 mg ● Carbohydrate 38.6 g ● Dietary Fiber 9.7 g ● Sugars 3.6 g ● Protein 7.0 g

Exchanges: 2 starch, 1 vegetable, 1 1/2 fat

Toasted Walnut Couscous

4 tablespoons tomato paste
1 cup low-sodium organic vegetable broth ▮
1/3 cup whole-wheat couscous
1/4 cup walnut pieces
1/2 tablespoon olive oil

1. Preheat toaster oven or broiler.
2. Combine tomato paste and broth in a medium saucepan. Bring to a boil over high heat.
3. Remove from heat. Add couscous. Stir, cover, and let stand 5 minutes.
4. Place walnuts on a foil-lined baking tray, and toast in oven or toaster oven or under a broiler for 2–3 minutes.
5. Add olive oil to the couscous, and fluff with a fork to separate grains.
6. Spoon onto individual plates, sprinkle toasted walnuts on top, and serve.

Preparation time: 10 minutes ● Servings: 2

Calories 265 ● Calories from Fat 122 ● Total Fat 13.6 g ● Saturated Fat 1.4 g ● Monounsaturated Fat 3.8 g ● Cholesterol 0 mg ● Sodium 310 mg ● Carbohydrate 33.1 g ● Dietary Fiber 4.9 g ● Sugars 5.8 g ● Protein 7.6 g

Exchanges: 2 starch, 2 1/2 fat

HELPFUL HINTS:

■ The bulgur wheat needs to soak for 20 minutes. While it soaks, prepare the rest of the meal.

■ Chop fresh herbs in a food processor.

■ Toast walnuts in a toaster oven or under a broiler. Watch them if under a broiler. They will burn easily.

SHOPPING LIST

Grocery
1 package fine bulgur wheat
1 package whole-wheat couscous
1 bottle lemon juice
1 can sliced black olives
1 small can tomato paste
1 can low-sodium organic vegetable broth ▮
1 package walnut pieces

Produce
1 bunch scallions
1 bunch flat leaf parsley
1 bunch mint
1 ripe medium tomato

Staples
Olive oil
Salt
Black peppercorns

▮ SHOP SMART!

Low-sodium organic vegetable broth (per cup): 12 calories, 3.0 g carbohydrate, 550 mg sodium

MUSHROOM PESTO PASTA WITH PIMENTO SALAD

Pesto is an uncooked sauce made with fresh basil, parsley, olive oil, and Parmesan cheese. It originated in Genoa, Italy.

Sauté some meaty Portobello mushrooms, and add them to the pesto to complete this flavorful pasta dish in the time it takes to boil pasta. Portobellos add a hearty flavor.

Mushroom Pesto Pasta

1/2 tablespoon olive oil
1/4 pound Portobello mushrooms, thinly sliced (2 cups)
1/4 cup reduced-fat prepared pesto sauce 🔲

1 tablespoon pine nuts
1/4 pound fresh linguine
Salt and freshly ground black pepper

COUNTDOWN

■ Put water for pasta on to boil.
■ Make Mushroom Pesto Pasta.
■ Make salad.

1. Bring 3–4 quarts of water to a boil in a large pot.
2. Heat the oil in a small nonstick skillet over medium-high heat. Sauté mushrooms for 5 minutes. Remove from skillet and chop.
3. Place mushrooms in a bowl. Add pesto sauce and pine nuts. Mix well.
4. Cook the linguine in the boiling water for 3 minutes or until it's cooked but still firm. Drain, and toss with the pesto sauce. Add salt and pepper to taste and serve.

Preparation time: 15 minutes ● Servings: 2

Calories 441 ● Calories from Fat 145 ● Total Fat 16.2 g ● Saturated Fat 3.0 g ● Monounsaturated Fat 9.4 g ● Cholesterol 8 mg ● Sodium 277 mg ● Carbohydrate 50.0 g ● Dietary Fiber 3.7 g ● Sugars 4.0 g ● Protein 14.1 g

Exchanges: 3 starch, 1 vegetable, 1 lean meat, 3 fat

Pimento Pepper Salad

4 cups washed ready-to-eat Italian-style salad
1 cup canned sweet pimento, drained and sliced
2 teaspoons olive oil
2 teaspoons balsamic vinegar
Salt and freshly ground black pepper

1. Arrange salad leaves on two dinner plates. In a small bowl, mix pimento, olive oil, and vinegar together. Add salt and pepper to taste.

2. Spoon over lettuce and serve.

Preparation time: 5 minutes ● Servings: 2

Calories 83 ● Calories from Fat 46 ● Total Fat 5.1 g ● Saturated Fat 0.7 g ● Monounsaturated Fat 3.3 g ● Cholesterol 0 mg ● Sodium 23 mg ● Carbohydrate 8.9 g ● Dietary Fiber 3.8 g ● Sugars 4.5 g ● Protein 2.2 g

Exchanges: 2 vegetable, 1 fat

HELPFUL HINTS:

■ Mushrooms can be chopped in a food processor.

■ Any type of washed lettuce can be used for the salad base.

SHOPPING LIST

Grocery
1 container reduced-fat pesto sauce ▯
1 package pine nuts
1/4 pound fresh linguine
1 jar/can sweet pimentos

Produce
1/4 pound Portobello mushrooms
1 bag washed ready-to-eat Italian-style salad

Staples
Olive oil
Balsamic vinegar
Salt
Black peppercorns

SHOP SMART!

Reduced-fat pesto sauce (per tablespoon): 80 calories, 4.8 total fat, 1.0 g saturated fat, 135 mg sodium [*Example*: Buitoni Reduced-Fat Pesto with Basil]

Index

Aga Khan's Chicken Curry, 88
Alcohol
Rum
Jerk Shrimp, 68
Vermouth
Crab Scampi, 82
Dijon Chicken, 118
Tarragon Chicken, 144
Whiskey
Whiskey Pork, 196
Whiskey-Soused Salmon, 22
Almond-Crusted Trout, 26
Almond-Grape Chicken Salad, 90
Apples
Aga Khan's Chicken Curry, 88
Brandied Apples and Pork, 162
Meatball, Beer, and Potato Stew, 210
Mulligatawny Soup, 258
Pork Chops with Apple Relish, 180
Turkey and Apple Salad, 148
Turkey Normandy, 150
Arroz con Jitomate (Rice with Tomato), 28
Arugula
Arugula Pasta, 9
Pan-Fried Pork with Garlic Greens, 178
Arugula Pasta, 9
Asparagus Rice, 25

Balsamic Grilled Tuna, 8
Balsamic Pork Scaloppini, 158
Barley
Barley and Broccoli Rabe, 183
Quick Barley, 237
Southwestern Barley Salad, 97

Barley and Broccoli Rabe, 183
Basque Chicken, 92
Beans
Black
Black Bean and Tomato Salad, 67
Black Bean Chicken Chili, 94
Cannellini
Country Mushroom and Sausage Soup, 112
Fennel and Bean Salad, 99
Garlic Rosemary Beans, 209
Pollo Tonnato (Chicken in Tuna Sauce), 140
Edamame
Frittata Primavera, 252
Lentils Vinaigrette, 71
Shrimp Caesar Salad, 74
Southwestern Three-Bean Soup, 262
Great Northern
Pimento Endive Salad, 73
Green
Aga Khan's Chicken Curry, 88
Beef in Oyster Sauce, 200
Green Bean Pimento Rice, 143
Lentils
Ham and Lentil Soup, 174
Lamb and Lentil Tagine, 246
Lentils and Rice, 257
Mulligatawny Soup, 258
Rosemary Lentils, 197
Lima
Hot Pepper Succotash, 47
Salmon, Quinoa, and Corn Salad, 14
Southwestern Three-Bean Soup, 262
Pinto
Pinto Bean Salad, 63

Refried
 Chicken Tostadas, 100
Sprouts
 Braised Chinese Shrimp, 54
 Chinese Noodles and Sprouts, 43

Beef
Buffalo Steak
 Walnut-Crusted Buffalo Steak, 230
Ground Beef
 Meatball, Beer, and Potato Stew, 210
 Spaghetti Bolognese (Spaghetti and Meat
  Sauce), 226
Ground Buffalo
 Buffalo Cheeseburgers, 202
Roast Beef
 Mock Hungarian Goulash, 214
 Roast Beef Chopped Salad, 220
 Roast Beef Hash, 222
 Roast Beef Pita Pocket with Tomato and
  Onion Relish, 224
Steak
 Beef in Oyster Sauce, 200
 Filet Marchand de Vin (Steak in Red Wine
  Sauce), 204
 Garlic Steak, 206
 Honey-Mustard Crusted Steak, 208
 Mediterranean Steak, 212
 Pan-Fried Ropa Vieja (Flank Steak in Tomato
  Sauce), 216
 Pistachio-Crusted Beef and Mixed Vegetable
  Kabobs, 218
 Steak and Portobello Sandwich, 228
 Vietnamese Hot and Spicy Stir-Fry Beef, 232
Beef in Oyster Sauce, 200
Beer-Soused Pork with Potato and Leeks, 160
Bell Peppers
 Five-Spice Pork and Rice Stir-Fry, 172
 Red Pepper and Tomato Penne, 171

Green
 Arroz con Jitomate (Rice with Tomato), 29
 Curried Chicken Pot Pie, 116
 Fried Corn and Green Pepper, 51
 Frittata Primavera, 252
 Greek Summer Salad, 225
 Meatball, Beer, and Potato Stew, 210
 Mock Hungarian Goulash, 214
 Pan-Fried Ropa Vieja (Flank Steak in Tomato
  Sauce), 216
 Roast Beef Chopped Salad, 220
 Sweet and Sour Shrimp, 56
 Thai Chicken Kabobs, 146
 Turkey Picadillo, 152
Red
 Chicken and Shiitake Yakitori, 104
 Chinese Salad with Asian Dressing, 108
 Pistachio-Crusted Beef and Mixed Vegetable
  Kabobs, 218
 Pollo Tonnato (Chicken in Tuna Sauce), 140
 Spicy Shrimp and Peach Salad, 70
 Vegetable Medley Rice, 77
Black Bean and Tomato Salad, 67
Black Bean Chicken Chili, 94
Black Bean Soup with Shrimp, 64
Bok Choy
 Ginger-Teriyaki Steamed Fish and Chinese
  Noodles, 36
 Stir-Fried Bok Choy and Noodles, 169
Braised Chinese Shrimp, 54
Brandied Apples and Pork, 162
Broccoli
 Broccoli and Potatoes, 23
 Broccoli and Sweet Potatoes, 193
 Broccoli Farfalle, 137
 Broccoli Linguine, 31
 Broccoli Rice Pilaf, 245
 Veal and Olive Stew, 236
 Vegetable Fettuccini, 19
 Vegetable Quinoa, 119

Broccoli Rabe
  Barley and Broccoli Rabe, 183
  Broccoli and Potatoes, 23
Broccoli and Sweet Potatoes, 193
Broccoli Farfalle, 137
Broccoli Linguine, 31
Broccoli Rice Pilaf, 245
Broth
  Chicken
    Black Bean Soup with Shrimp, 64
    Broccoli Rice Pilaf, 245
    Coq au Vin (Chicken Stewed in Red Wine), 110
    Country Mushroom and Sausage Soup, 112
    Cucumber Rice Salad, 139
    Curried Chicken Pot Pie, 116
    Filet Marchand de Vin (Steak in Red Wine Sauce), 204
    Fish in a Pouch, 34
    Five-Spice Pork and Rice Stir-Fry, 172
    Garlic Rosemary Beans, 209
    Meatball, Beer, and Potato Stew, 210
    Poached Chicken with Fresh Tomato Mayonnaise Sauce, 138
    Pork in Port Wine, 182
    Rice and Peas, 69
    Roast Beef Hash, 222
    Sautéed Garlic Potatoes, 205
    Tarragon Chicken, 144
    Turkey Stroganoff, 154
  Vegetable
    Greek-Style Casserole Soup, 254
    Mulligatawny Soup, 258
    Toasted Walnut Couscous, 265
Brown Rice, 57, 111, 147, 153, 217
Buffalo Cheeseburgers, 202

Cabbage
  Braised Chinese Shrimp, 54
  Jalapeño Coleslaw, 11

Cajun-Bronzed Mahi-Mahi, 38
Capers
  Pollo Tonnato (Chicken in Tuna Sauce), 140
  Turkey Picadillo, 152
  Veal Milanese, 242
Caraway Noodles, 215
Carrots
  Carrots and Rice, 79
  Coq au Vin (Chicken Stewed in Red Wine), 110
  Mulligatawny Soup, 258
  Pan-Fried Ropa Vieja (Flank Steak in Tomato Sauce), 216
  Pecan Spinach Salad, 13
  Ricotta Soufflé, 260
  Roast Beef Chopped Salad, 220
  Tarragon Chicken, 144
  Vegetable Fettuccini, 19
  Zucchini Carrot Gratinée, 129
Carrots and Rice, 79
Celery
  Celery and Fennel Salad, 59
  Celery with Blue Cheese Dressing, 125
  Coq au Vin (Chicken Stewed in Red Wine), 110
  Fish Chowder, 48
  Greek-Style Casserole Soup, 254
  Mulligatawny Soup, 258
  Roast Beef Chopped Salad, 220
  Spaghetti Bolognese (Spaghetti and Meat Sauce), 226
Cheese
  Cheddar
    Buffalo Cheeseburgers, 202
    Shrimp Mushroom Quesadillas, 66
  Feta
    Greek Salad, 187
    Greek-Style Casserole Soup, 254
  Goat
    Herbed Cheese Crostini, 149

Mexican-Style
  Black Bean Chicken Chili, 94
  Mexican Sopes (Layered Open Tortilla
    Sandwich), 134
  Southwestern Three-Bean Soup, 262
Parmesan
  Arugula Pasta, 9
  Curried Chicken Pot Pie, 116
  Gratinéed Fennel, 253
  Parmesan Corn, 121
  Parmesan Sole, 32
  Shrimp Caesar Salad, 74
  Tomato-Basil Pasta, 177
  Veal Milanese, 242
  Zucchini Carrot Gratinée, 129
Ricotta
  Ricotta Soufflé, 260
Chicken
  Aga Khan's Chicken Curry, 88
  Almond-Grape Chicken Salad, 90
  Basque Chicken, 92
  Black Bean Chicken Chili, 94
  Chicken and Garlic Greens, 102
  Chicken and Shiitake Yakitori, 104
  Chicken and Walnuts in Lettuce Puffs, 106
  Chicken Diavolo (Italian Chicken in Spicy
    Tomato Sauce), 128
  Chicken Pizzaioli, 98
  Chicken Tostadas, 100
  Chili Chicken, 96
  Chinese Salad with Asian Dressing, 108
  Coq au Vin (Chicken Stewed in Red Wine),
    110
  Crispy Chicken, 114
  Curried Chicken Pot Pie, 116
  Dijon Chicken, 118
  Grilled Chicken Wraps, 120
  Hawaiian Chicken, 122
  Honey-Spiced Mock Chicken Wings, 124
  Indian-Spiced Chicken, 126

Jacques Pepin's Supreme of Chicken with
    Balsamic Vinegar and Onion Sauce, 130
  Marsala-Glazed Chicken, 132
  Mexican Sopes (Layered Open Tortilla
    Sandwich), 134
  Pistachio-Crusted Chicken, 136
  Poached Chicken with Fresh Tomato
    Mayonnaise Sauce, 138
  Pollo Tonnato (Chicken in Tuna Sauce), 140
  Sherry Chicken, 142
  Tarragon Chicken, 144
  Thai Chicken Kabobs, 146
Chili Chicken, 96
Chili Pepper Potatoes, 207
Chilled Cucumber and Salmon Soup, 16
Chimichurri Pork Chops, 164
Chinese Noodles, 201
Chinese Noodles and Sprouts, 43
Chinese Noodles and Snow Peas, 233
Chinese Pan-Roasted Pork, 168
Chinese Pork Puffs, 166
Chinese Rice, 107
Chinese Salad with Asian Dressing, 108
Chipotle Corn and Zucchini, 45
Cilantro Tomatoes, 101
Coq au Vin (Chicken Stewed in Red Wine), 110
Corn
  Black Bean Chicken Chili, 94
  Chipotle Corn and Zucchini, 45
  Corn and Peas, 131
  Fried Corn and Green Pepper, 51
  Hot Pepper Succotash, 47
  Parmesan Corn, 121
  Pistachio-Crusted Beef and Mixed Vegetable
    Kabobs, 218
  Salmon, Quinoa, and Corn Salad, 14
  Southwestern Barley Salad, 97
Country Garlic Toast, 175
Country Mushroom and Sausage Soup, 112

Couscous
> Garlic Couscous, 35
> Lemon-Pepper Shrimp and Couscous on a
> > Bed of Spinach, 60
> Minted Couscous, 213
> Toasted Walnut Couscous, 265

Crab Scampi, 82
Crispy Chicken, 114
Crunchy Coleslaw, 91

Cucumbers
> Braised Chinese Shrimp, 54
> Chilled Cucumber and Salmon Soup, 16
> Chinese Pork Puffs, 166
> Cucumber Rice Salad, 139
> Greek Summer Salad, 225
> Middle-Eastern Lamb, 248
> Pork Pita Pocket, 186
> Quick-Fried Diced Veal, 238
> Salmon Gazpacho, 20

Cumin-Crusted Snapper, 28
Cumin-Scented Rice and Spinach, 127
Curried Chicken Pot Pie, 116
Curry-Kissed Scallops, 78

Dijon Chicken, 118
Dijon Pork, 170
Dilled Potatoes, 33

Egg Noodles, 155, 163

Fennel
> Celery and Fennel Salad, 59
> Fennel and Bean Salad, 99
> Gratinéed Fennel, 253

Filet Marchand de Vin (Steak in Red Wine Sauce),
204

Fish (*see also Salmon, Tilapia, Tuna*)
> Almond-Crusted Trout, 26
> Cajun Bronzed Mahi-Mahi, 38
> Cumin-Crusted Snapper, 28
> Fish Chowder, 48
> Fish in a Pouch, 34
> Ginger-Teriyaki Steamed Fish and Chinese
> > Noodles, 36
> Halibut in Cider, 40
> Mexican Orange Fillet, 50
> Parmesan Sole, 32
> Sicilian Swordfish, 30
> Spaghetti with Clams and Herb Sauce, 84

Five-Spice Fillet, 42
Five-Spice Pork, 172
Fresh Fettuccini, 81
Fresh Linguine, 191
Fried Corn and Green Pepper, 51
Frittata Primavera, 252

Garlic Couscous, 35
Garlic Rosemary Beans, 209
Garlic Steak, 206
Garlic Sweet Potatoes and Sugar Snap Peas, 159
Ginger-Teriyaki Steamed Fish and Chinese Noodles,
36
Gratinéed Fennel, 253
Greek Salad, 187
Greek-Style Casserole Soup, 254
Greek Summer Salad, 225
Green Bean Pimento Rice, 143
Green Salad, 49
Grilled Chicken Wraps, 120

Half and Half
> Curry-Kissed Scallops, 78
> Dijon Chicken, 118
> Fish Chowder, 48

Marsala-Glazed Chicken, 132
Tarragon Chicken, 144
Turkey Normandy, 150
Halibut in Cider, 40
Ham
    Basque Chicken, 92
    Coq au Vin (Chicken Stewed in Red Wine),
      110
    Fish Chowder, 48
    Ham and Lentil Soup, 174
Hawaiian Chicken, 122
Herbed Cheese Crostini, 149
Herbed Grilled Pork, 176
Herbed Zucchini, 227
Honey
    Braised Chinese Shrimp, 54
    Brandied Apples and Pork, 162
    Chicken and Shiitake Yakitori, 104
    Chinese Pan-Roasted Pork, 168
    Honey-Mustard Crusted Steak, 208
    Honey-Soy Glazed Salmon, 24
    Honey-Spiced Mock Chicken Wings, 124
    Pork Chops with Apple Relish, 180
    Pork Medallions with Red Berry Sauce, 184
    Southwestern Honey-Glazed Pork, 194
Hot Glazed Tuna Steak, 12
Hot Pepper Shrimp, 72
Hot Pepper Succotash, 47

Iceberg Salad, 95
Indian-Spiced Chicken, 126
Indian-Spiced Spinach, 256
Italian Salad, 85

Jacques Pepin's Supreme of Chicken with Balsamic
    Vinegar and Onion Sauce, 130
Jalapeño Coleslaw, 11

Jams and Jelly
    Apricot Jam
      Curry-Kissed Scallops, 78
    Hot Pepper Jelly
      Hot Pepper Succotash, 47
      Pistachio-Crusted Beef and Mixed Vegetable
        Kabobs, 218
      Walnut-Crusted Buffalo Steak, 230
    Orange Marmalade
      Hot Glazed Tuna Steak, 12
      Turkey and Apple Salad, 148
Jerk Shrimp, 68
Juice
    Apple
      Brandied Apples and Pork, 162
      Turkey Normandy, 150
    Clam
      Spaghetti with Clams and Herb Sauce, 84
    Cranberry
      Pork Medallions with Red Berry Sauce, 184
    Orange
      Mexican Orange Fillet, 50
      Veaux aux Oranges (Veal in Orange Sauce),
        244
    Pineapple
      Hawaiian Chicken, 122
    Tomato
      Fish Chowder, 48
      Lemon-Pepper Shrimp and Couscous on a
        Bed of Spinach, 60
      Salmon Gazpacho, 20
      Spinach Pilaf, 39

Lamb
    Lamb and Lentil Tagine, 246
    Middle-Eastern Lamb, 248
Leeks
    Beer-Soused Pork with Potato and Leeks, 160
    Turkey Normandy, 150

Lemon-Pepper Shrimp and Couscous on a Bed of
    Spinach, 60
Lentils and Rice, 257
Lentils Vinaigrette, 71
Lettuce
    Almond-Grape Chicken Salad, 90
    Chicken and Walnuts in Lettuce Puffs, 106
    Chicken Tostadas, 100
    Chili Chicken, 96
    Chinese Pork Puffs, 166
    Chinese Salad with Asian Dressing, 108
    Green Salad, 49
    Grilled Chicken Wraps, 120
    Iceberg Salad, 95
    Italian Salad, 85
    Mexican Sopes (Layered Open Tortilla
        Sandwich), 134
    Pineapple Salad, 123
    Pinto Bean Salad, 63
    Roast Beef Chopped Salad, 220
    Shrimp Caesar Salad, 74
    Spicy Shrimp and Peach Salad, 70
    Turkey and Apple Salad, 148
Linguine with Summer Squash, 189

Marsala-Glazed Chicken, 132
Mayonnaise
    Almond-Grape Chicken Salad, 90
    Crunchy Coleslaw, 91
    Dijon Pork, 170
    Jalapeño Coleslaw, 11
    Poached Chicken with Fresh Tomato
        Mayonnaise Sauce, 138
    Pollo Tonnato (Chicken in Tuna Sauce), 140
    Salsa Potato Salad, 195
    Spicy Shrimp and Peach Salad, 70
    Turkey and Apple Salad, 148
    Whiskey-Soused Salmon, 22
Meatball, Beer, and Potato Stew, 210

Mediterranean Steak, 212
Mexican Orange Fillet, 50
Mexican Sope (Layered Open Tortilla Sandwich),
    134
Middle-Eastern Lamb, 248
Minted Couscous, 213
Mixed Green Salad, 49, 223
Mixed Salad, 203
Mixed-Herb Angel Hair Pasta, 185
Mock Hungarian Goulash, 214
Mulligatawny Soup, 258
Mushroom Pesto Pasta, 266
Mushrooms
    Filet Marchand de Vin (Steak in Red Wine
        Sauce), 204
    Vegetable Medley Rice, 77
    Baby Bello
        Curried Chicken Pot Pie, 116
        Fish in a Pouch, 34
        Frittata Primavera, 252
        Pistachio-Crusted Beef and Mixed Vegetable
            Kabobs, 218
        Shrimp Mushroom Quesadillas, 66
    Button
        Coq au Vin (Chicken Stewed in Red Wine),
            110
        Country Mushroom and Sausage Soup, 112
        Garlic Steak, 206
        Jacques Pepin's Supreme of Chicken with
            Balsamic Vinegar and Onion Sauce, 130
        Ratatouille, 115
        Ricotta Soufflé, 260
        Turkey Stroganoff, 154
    Portobello
        Mock Hungarian Goulash, 214
        Mushroom Pesto Pasta, 266
        Steak and Portobello Sandwich, 228
    Shiitake
        Chicken and Shiitake Yakitori, 104
        Chicken and Walnuts in Lettuce Puffs, 106

Chinese Salad with Asian Dressing, 108
Roast Beef Hash, 222

Mustard

Dijon

Dijon Chicken, 118
Dijon Pork, 170
Hawaiian Chicken, 122
Hot Glazed Tuna Steak, 12
Spicy Shrimp and Peach Salad, 70
Turkey Stroganoff, 154
Whiskey Pork, 196

Honey

Honey-Mustard Crusted Steak, 208

Nuts

Almonds

Almond-Crusted Trout, 26
Almond-Grape Chicken Salad, 90
Braised Chinese Shrimp, 54
Five-Spice Pork and Rice Stir-Fry, 172
Mulligatawny Soup, 258

Cashews

Chinese Salad with Asian Dressing, 108

Macadamia Nuts

Pineapple Salad, 123

Pecans

Pecan Spinach Salad, 13
Pecan-Crusted Tilapia, 46

Pine Nuts

Indian-Spiced Spinach, 256
Mushroom Pesto Pasta, 266
Pesto Scallops, 80
Roast Beef Hash, 222

Pistachios

Greek-Style Casserole Soup, 254
Pistachio-Crusted Beef and Mixed Vegetable
    Kabobs, 218
Pistachio-Crusted Chicken, 136

Walnuts

Beef in Oyster Sauce, 200
Chicken and Walnuts in Lettuce Puffs, 106
Mediterranean Steak, 212
Shrimp Caesar Salad, 74
Toasted Walnut Couscous, 265
Vietnamese Hot and Spicy Stir-Fry Beef, 232
Walnut-Crusted Buffalo Steak, 230
Zucchini Carrot Gratinée, 129

Oil, Sesame

Beef in Oyster Sauce, 200
Braised Chinese Shrimp, 54
Chicken and Walnuts in Lettuce Puffs, 106
Chinese Noodles and Snow Peas, 233
Chinese Noodles and Sprouts, 43
Chinese Pan-Roasted Pork, 168
Chinese Pork Puffs, 166
Chinese Rice, 107
Chinese Salad with Asian Dressing, 108
Five-Spice Fillet, 42
Quick Stir-Fried Rice, 167
Quick-Fried Diced Veal, 238
Sesame Rice, 105
Simple Fried Rice, 239
Stir-Fried Bok Choy and Noodles, 169

Olives

Chicken Pizzaioli, 98
Greek Summer Salad, 225
Mediterranean Steak, 212
Pollo Tonnato (Chicken in Tuna Sauce), 140
Sicilian Swordfish, 30
Tabbouleh, 264
Veal and Olive Stew, 236

Onion-Garlic Crostini, 113

Orzo

Orzo and Chives, 145
Roman Spinach, 133

Pan-Fried Pork with Garlic Greens, 178
Pan-Fried Ropa Vieja (Flank Steak in Tomato Sauce), 216
Pan-Seared Scallops, 76
Parmesan Corn, 121
Parmesan Sole, 32
Pasta
  Angel Hair
    Mixed-Herb Angel Hair Pasta, 185
  Farfalle
    Broccoli Farfalle, 137
  Fettuccini
    Arugula Pasta, 9
    Fresh Fettuccini, 81
    Vegetable Fettuccini, 19
  Linguine
    Broccoli Linguine, 31
    Linguine with Summer Squash, 189
    Mushroom Pesto Pasta, 266
    Salsa Pork with Fresh Linguine, 190
    Tomato-Basil Pasta, 177
  Noodles
    Caraway Noodles, 215
    Chinese Noodles, 201
    Chinese Noodles and Snow Peas, 233
    Chinese Noodles and Sprouts, 43
    Chinese Salad with Asian Dressing, 108
    Egg Noodles, 155, 163
    Ginger-Teriyaki Steamed Fish and Chinese Noodles, 36
    Stir-Fried Bok Choy and Noodles, 169
  Penne
    Penne ala Sicialianna (Sicilian Penne Pasta), 241
    Penne and Sugar Snap Peas, 27
    Red Pepper and Tomato Penne, 171
    Shrimp Caesar Salad, 74
  Spaghetti
    Spaghetti Bolognese (Spaghetti and Meat Sauce), 226

Spaghetti del Pescatore (Fisherman's Spaghetti), 58
    Spaghetti with Clams and Herb Sauce, 84
    Spaghetti, 83
  Spaghettini
    Spaghetti Pomodoro, 243
Pecan Spinach Salad, 13
Pecan-Crusted Tilapia, 46
Penne ala Siciliana (Sicilian Penne Pasta), 241
Peas
  Chinese Noodles and Snow Peas, 233
  Corn and Peas, 131
  Curried Chicken Pot Pie, 116
  Garlic Sweet Potatoes and Sugar Snap Peas, 159
  Penne and Sugar Snap Peas, 25
  Rice and Peas, 69
  Salsa Pork with Fresh Linguine, 190
  Simple Fried Rice, 239
  Spicy Shrimp and Peach Salad, 70
Peppers *(see also Bell Peppers)*
  Jalapeño
    Jalapeño Coleslaw, 11
    Rice and Peas, 69
  Poblano
    Chili Pepper Potatoes, 207
    Poblano Rice, 53
    Shrimp and Poblano Pepper Tacos, 62
  Pimento
    Basque Chicken, 92
    Green Bean Pimento Rice, 143
    Pan-Fried Ropa Vieja (Flank Steak in Tomato Sauce), 216
    Pimento Endive Salad, 73
    Pimento Pepper Salad, 267
    Roast Beef Hash, 222
Pesto Scallops, 80
Pimento Endive Salad, 73
Pimento Pepper Salad, 267

Pineapple
  Pineapple Salad, 123
  Sautéed Fish with Pineapple Salsa, 52
Pinto Bean Salad, 63
Pistachio-Crusted Beef and Vegetable Kabobs, 218
Pistachio-Crusted Chicken, 136
Poached Chicken with Fresh Tomato Mayonnaise
    Sauce, 138
Poached Salmon with Chive Sauce, 18
Poblano Rice, 53
Pollo Tonnato (Chicken in Tuna Sauce), 140
Pork
  Balsamic Pork Scaloppini, 158
  Beer-Soused Pork with Potato and Leeks, 160
  Brandied Apples and Pork, 162
  Chimichurri Pork Chops, 164
  Chinese Pan-Roasted Pork, 168
  Chinese Pork Puffs, 166
  Dijon Pork, 170
  Five-Spice Pork and Rice Stir-Fry, 172
  Herbed Grilled Pork, 176
  Pan-Fried Pork with Garlic Greens, 178
  Pork Chops with Apple Relish, 180
  Pork in Port Wine, 182
  Pork Medallions with Red Berry Sauce, 184
  Pork Pita Pocket, 186
  Pork with Chunky Strawberry Salsa, 188
  Salsa Pork with Fresh Linguine, 190
  Sara Moulton's Pork Scaloppini, 192
  Southwestern Honey-Glazed Pork, 194
  Whiskey Pork, 196
Pork Chops with Apple Relish, 180
Pork in Port Wine, 182
Pork Medallions with Red Berry Sauce, 184
Pork Pita Pocket, 186
Potatoes
  Beer-Soused Pork with Potato and Leeks, 160
  Broccoli and Potatoes, 23
  Dilled Potatoes, 33
  Fish Chowder, 48

  Roast Beef Hash, 222
  Sautéed Garlic Potatoes, 205
  Spicy Sautéed Potatoes, 103
Red
  Chili Pepper Potatoes, 207
  Frittata Primavera, 252
  Salsa Potato Salad, 195
  Spicy Roast Potatoes, 179
Sweet Potatoes
  Broccoli and Sweet Potatoes, 193
  Garlic Sweet Potatoes and Sugar Snap Peas,
    159
  Meatball, Beer, and Potato Stew, 210
  Sweet Potatoes, 151, 181

Quick Barley, 237
Quick-Fried Diced Veal, 238
Quick Rice and Tomatoes, 165
Quick Stir-Fried Rice, 167
Quinoa
  Salmon, Quinoa, and Corn Salad, 14
  Vegetable Quinoa, 119

Ratatouille (Sautéed Provençal Vegetables), 115
Red Pepper and Tomato Penne, 171
Rice, 89
Rice
Arborio
  Greek-Style Casserole Soup, 254
Basmati
  Cumin-Scented Rice and Spinach, 127
Brown
  Arroz con Jitomate (Rice with Tomato), 29
  Asparagus Rice, 25
  Brown Rice, 57, 111, 147, 153, 217
  Carrots and Rice, 79
  Cucumber Rice Salad, 139
  Five-Spice Pork and Rice Stir-Fry, 172

Lentils and Rice, 257
Poblano Rice, 53
Quick Stir-Fried Rice, 167
Saffron Rice, 41
Sesame Rice, 105
Simple Fried Rice, 239
Spinach Brown Rice, 249
Vegetable Medley Rice, 77
White
    Broccoli Rice Pilaf, 245
    Chinese Rice, 107
    Green Bean Pimento Rice, 143
    Quick Rice and Tomatoes, 165
    Rice and Peas, 69
    Rice, 89
    Rice and Spinach Pilaf, 39
Ricotta Soufflé, 260
Roast Beef Chopped Salad, 220
Roast Beef Hash, 222
Roast Beef Pita Pocket with Tomato and Onion
    Relish, 224
Roast Pork with Chunky Strawberry Salsa, 188
Roman Spinach, 133
Rosemary Lentils, 197

Saffron Rice, 41, 92
Salmon
    Chilled Cucumber and Salmon Soup, 16
    Honey-Soy Glazed Salmon, 24
    Poached Salmon with Chive Sauce, 18
    Salmon Gazpacho, 20
    Salmon, Quinoa, and Corn Salad, 14
    Whiskey-Soused Salmon, 22
Salsa
    Mexican Sopes (Layered Open Tortilla
        Sandwich), 134
    Salsa Pork with Fresh Linguine, 190
    Salsa Potato Salad, 195

Sautéed Fish with Pineapple Salsa, 52
Southwestern Barley Salad, 97
Sara Moulton's Pork Scaloppini, 192
Sauces
Barbecue
    Grilled Chicken Wraps, 120
Hot Pepper
    Basque Chicken, 92
    Black Bean Soup with Shrimp, 64
    Chicken Pizzaioli, 98
    Crab Scampi, 82
    Fried Corn and Green Pepper, 51
    Pork with Chunky Strawberry Salsa, 188
    Vietnamese Hot and Spicy Stir-Fry Beef, 232
Oyster
    Beef in Oyster Sauce, 200
    Chicken and Walnuts in Lettuce Puffs, 106
Pasta
    Chicken Diavolo (Italian Chicken in Spicy
        Tomato Sauce), 128
    Chicken Pizzaioli, 98
    Country Mushroom and Sausage Soup, 112
    Hawaiian Chicken, 122
    Mock Hungarian Goulash, 214
    Ratatouille, 115
Pesto
    Mushroom Pesto Pasta, 266
    Pesto Scallops, 80
Sweet and Sour
    Sweet and Sour Shrimp, 56
Soy
    Braised Chinese Shrimp, 54
    Chinese Pan-Roasted Pork, 168
    Chinese Salad with Asian Dressing, 108
    Five-Spice Fillet, 42
    Five-Spice Pork and Rice Stir-Fry, 172
    Honey-Soy Glazed Salmon, 24
    Quick-Fried Diced Veal, 238
    Southwestern Honey-Glazed Pork, 194
    Stir-Fried Bok Choy and Noodles, 169

Teriyaki
  Chicken and Shiitake Yakitori, 104
  Ginger-Teriyaki Steamed Fish and Chinese
      Noodles, 36
Thai Peanut
  Thai Chicken Kabobs, 146
Tomato
  Spaghetti del Pescatore (Fisherman's
      Spaghetti), 58
  Turkey Picadillo, 152
Worcestershire
  Crab Scampi, 82
  Turkey Picadillo, 152
Sautéed Fish with Pineapple Salsa, 52
Sautéed Garlic Potatoes, 205
Scallops
  Curry-Kissed Scallops, 78
  Pan-Seared Scallops, 76
  Pesto Scallops, 80
Scaloppini al Marsala (Veal Marsala), 240
Seasonings
Chili Powder
  Black Bean Chicken Chili, 94
  Chili Chicken, 96
  Southwestern Three-Bean Soup, 262
Chinese
  Five Spice Fillet, 42
  Five-Spice Pork and Rice Stir-Fry, 172
Chipotle
  Chipotle Corn and Zucchini, 45
  Southwestern Fish Fillet, 44
Jerk
  Jerk Shrimp, 68
Sesame Rice, 105
Sherry Chicken, 142
Shrimp
  Black Bean Soup with Shrimp, 64
  Braised Chinese Shrimp, 54
  Hot Pepper Shrimp, 72
  Jerk Shrimp, 68

Lemon-Pepper Shrimp and Couscous on a
    Bed of Spinach, 60
Shrimp and Poblano Pepper Tacos, 62
Shrimp Caesar Salad, 74
Shrimp Mushroom Quesadillas, 66
Spaghetti del Pescatore (Fisherman's
    Spaghetti), 58
Spicy Shrimp and Peach Salad, 70
Sweet and Sour Shrimp, 56
Sicilian Swordfish, 30
Simple Fried Rice, 239
Sour Cream
  Chicken Tostadas, 100
  Mock Hungarian Goulash, 214
  Turkey Stroganoff, 154
Southwestern Barley Salad, 97
Southwestern Fish Fillet, 44
Southwestern Honey-Glazed Pork, 194
Southwestern Three-Bean Soup, 262
Spaghetti, 83
Spaghetti Bolognese (Spaghetti and Meat Sauce),
    226
Spaghetti del Pescatore (Fisherman's Spaghetti), 58
Spaghetti with Clams and Herb Sauce, 84
Spaghettini Pomodoro, 243
Spicy Roast Potatoes, 179
Spicy Sautéed Potatoes, 103
Spicy Shrimp and Peach Salad, 70
Spinach
  Chili Pepper Potatoes, 207
  Cumin-Scented Rice and Spinach, 127
  Greek-Style Casserole Soup, 254
  Indian-Spiced Spinach, 256
  Lamb and Lentil Tagine, 246
  Lemon-Pepper Shrimp and Couscous on a
      Bed of Spinach, 60
  Pecan Spinach Salad, 13
  Roman Spinach, 133
  Salmon, Quinoa, and Corn Salad, 14
  Shrimp Mushroom Quesadillas, 66

Spinach Brown Rice, 249
Spinach Pilaf, 39
Squash, Yellow
    Linguine with Summer Squash, 189
    Thai Chicken Kabobs, 146
Steak and Portobello Sandwich, 228
Stir-Fried Bok Choy and Noodles, 169
Sugar Snap Peas, 159
Sweet and Sour Shrimp, 56
Sweet Potatoes, 151, 181

Tabbouleh, 264
Tapenade-Topped Tomatoes, 229
Tarragon Chicken, 144
Texas Tuna Burger, 10
Thai Chicken Kabobs, 146
Tilapia
    Fish Chowder, 48
    Five-Spice Fillet, 42
    Pecan-Crusted Tilapia, 46
    Sautéed Fish with Pineapple Salsa, 52
    Southwestern Fish Fillet, 44
Toasted Walnut Couscous, 265
Tomatoes
    Aga Khan's Chicken Curry, 88
    Arroz con Jitomate (Rice with Tomato), 29
    Basque Chicken, 92
    Black Bean and Tomato Salad, 67
    Black Bean Chicken Chili, 94
    Black Bean Soup with Shrimp, 64
    Chili Chicken, 96
    Cilantro Tomatoes, 101
    Coq au Vin (Chicken Stewed in Red Wine), 110
    Crab Scampi, 82
    Fresh Fettuccini, 81
    Greek-Style Casserole Soup, 254
    Grilled Chicken Wraps, 120
    Halibut in Cider, 40

Ham and Lentil Soup, 174
Indian-Spiced Spinach, 256
Jerk Shrimp, 68
Lamb and Lentil Tagine, 246
Meatball, Beer, and Potato Stew, 210
Minted Couscous, 213
Mock Hungarian Goulash, 214
Pan-Fried Ropa Vieja (Flank Steak in Tomato Sauce), 216
Parmesan Sole, 32
Pinto Bean Salad, 63
Poached Chicken with Fresh Tomato Mayonnaise Sauce, 138
Quick Rice and Tomatoes, 165
Red Pepper and Tomato Penne, 171
Roast Beef Pita Pocket with Tomato and Onion Relish, 224
Salmon Gazpacho, 20
Salmon, Quinoa, and Corn Salad, 14
Sara Moulton's Pork Scaloppini, 192
Sicilian Swordfish, 30
Southwestern Three-Bean Soup, 262
Spaghetti Bolognese (Spaghetti and Meat Sauce), 226
Spaghetti Pomodoro, 243
Spaghetti with Clams and Herb Sauce, 84
Sweet and Sour Shrimp, 56
Tabbouleh, 264
Tapenade-Topped Tomatoes, 229
Tomato and Bean Salad, 231
Veal and Olive Stew, 236
Cherry
    Greek Salad, 187
    Thai Chicken Kabobs, 146
    Tomato Bruschetta, 261
Paste
    Toasted Walnut Couscous, 265
    Tomato-Basil Pasta, 177
    Turkey Stroganoff, 154
    Vietnamese Hot and Spicy Stir-Fry Beef, 232

Plum
Tomato-Basil Pasta, 177
Sun-Dried
Fish in a Pouch, 34
Tortillas
Chicken Tostadas, 100
Grilled Chicken Wraps, 120
Mexican Sopes (Layered Open Tortilla
Sandwich), 134
Shrimp and Poblano Pepper Tacos, 62
Shrimp Mushroom Quesadillas, 66
Chips
Fried Corn and Green Pepper, 51
Tuna
Balsamic Grilled Tuna, 8
Hot Glazed Tuna Steak, 12
Pollo Tonnato (Chicken in Tuna Sauce), 140
Texas Tuna Burger, 10
Turkey
Country Mushroom and Sausage Soup, 112
Turkey and Apple Salad, 148
Turkey Normandy, 150
Turkey Picadillo, 152
Turkey Stroganoff, 154
Veal
Quick-Fried Diced Veal, 238
Scaloppini al Marsala (Veal Marsala), 240
Veal and Olive Stew, 236
Veal Milanese, 242
Veaux aux Oranges (Veal in Orange Sauce),
244
Vegetable Fettuccini, 19
Vegetable Medley Rice, 77
Vegetable Quinoa, 119
Vietnamese Hot and Spicy Stir-Fry Beef, 232
Vinegar
Apple Cider
Pork Chops with Apple Relish, 180

Balsamic
Balsamic Grilled Tuna, 8
Balsamic Pork Scaloppini, 158
Chicken and Garlic Greens, 102
Ham and Lentil Soup, 174
Pimento Pepper Salad, 267
Roast Beef Pita Pocket with Tomato and
Onion Relish, 224
Salmon Gazpacho, 20
Steak and Portobello Sandwich, 228
Cider
Beer-Soused Pork with Potato and Leeks, 160
Mixed-Herb Angel Hair Pasta, 185
Pork Medallions with Red Berry Sauce, 184
Red Wine
Chicken and Shiitake Yakitori, 104
White
Crunchy Coleslaw, 91
Honey-Spiced Mock Chicken Wings, 124
Turkey Picadillo, 152

Walnut-Crusted Buffalo Steak, 230
Whiskey Pork, 196
Whiskey-Soused Salmon, 22
Wine
Marsala
Marsala-Glazed Chicken, 132
Scaloppini al Marsala (Veal Marsala), 240
Port
Pork in Port Wine, 182
Red
Coq au Vin (Chicken Stewed in Red Wine),
110
Sherry
Braised Chinese Shrimp, 54
Sherry Chicken, 142
Veaux aux Oranges (Veal in Orange Sauce),
244

Yogurt
 Almond-Grape Chicken Salad, 90
 Chilled Cucumber and Salmon Soup, 16
 Dijon Pork, 170
 Indian-Spiced Chicken, 126
 Middle-Eastern Lamb, 248
 Pollo Tonnato (Chicken in Tuna Sauce), 140
 Pork Pita Pocket, 186
 Salmon Gazpacho, 20
 Salsa Potato Salad, 195
 Turkey and Apple Salad, 148
 Vegetable Medley Rice, 77

Zucchini
 Chipotle Corn and Zucchini, 45
 Greek-Style Casserole Soup, 254
 Herbed Zucchini, 227
 Ratatouille, 115
 Ricotta Soufflé, 260
 Zucchini Carrot Gratinée, 129

Other Titles from the American Diabetes Association

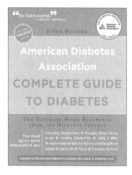

American Diabetes Association Complete Guide to Diabetes, 5th Edition
by American Diabetes Association

Have all of the tips and information on diabetes that you need close at hand. Complete with diagrams and easy-to-understand illustrations, sample medical forms, and an extensive list of resources, this guide breaks down how to live well with diabetes. The world's largest collection of diabetes self-care tips, techniques, and solutions to diabetes-related problems is back in its fifth edition, and it's bigger and better than ever before.

Order no. 4809-05; Price $22.95

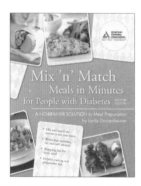

Mix 'n' Match Meals in Minutes for People with Diabetes, 2nd Edition
by Linda Gassenheimer

Designed for simplicity and diversity, *Mix 'n' Match Meals in Minutes* offers an assortment of breakfast, lunch, and dinner recipes for people who need entire meals in a snap. In this edition, you'll find an all-new section on speed meals that spice up any meal plan with healthy and hearty meals you can prepare in mere minutes. Don't settle for flavorless foods just because you're busy!

Order no. 4644-02; Price $16.95

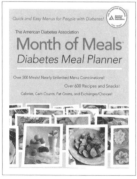

American Diabetes Association Month of Meals Diabetes Meal Planner
by American Diabetes Association

The bestselling Month of Meals™ series is all here—newly updated and collected into one complete, authoritative volume! Forget about the hassle of planning meals and spending hours making menus fit your diabetes management. With this invaluable guide, you'll have millions of daily menu combinations at your fingertips. Simply pick a menu for each meal, prepare your recipes, and enjoy a full day of delicious meals tailored specifically to you. It's as easy as that!

Order no. 4679-01; Price $22.95

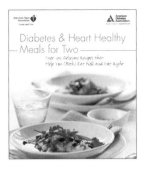

Diabetes & Heart Healthy Meals for Two

by the American Diabetes Association and the American Heart Association

If you or a loved one has diabetes, you need to eat heart-healthy meals. The simple, flavorful recipes were designed for those looking to improve or maintain their cardiovascular health. Each recipe is for two people, making this book perfect for adults without children in the house or for those who want to keep leftovers to a minimum. With over 170 recipes, there are countless options to keep your heart at its healthiest and your blood glucose under control.

Order no. 4673-01; Price $18.95

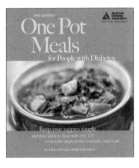

One Pot Meals for People with Diabetes, 2nd Edition

by Ruth Glick and Nancy Baggett

Nothing is easier than "one-pot" cooking—prepare your ingredients, combine, and let them cook! Now in a new and improved second edition, create meals from pasta to casseroles to hearty sandwiches in a snap. Inside, you'll find choices to satisfy any appetite at any time!

Order no. 4635-02; Price $14.95

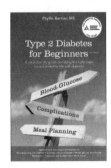

Type 2 Diabetes for Beginners, 2nd Edition

by Phillis Barrier, MS, RD, CDE

If you've recently been diagnosed with type 2 diabetes, this book is your road map to staying healthy. In this fully revised second edition, you'll get the latest information about living with type 2 diabetes and the answers to your questions about blood glucose levels, prevention of complications, and how meal planning keeps you balanced.

Order no. 4877-02; Price $14.95

To order these and other great American Diabetes Association titles, call **1-800-232-6733** or visit **http://shopdiabetes.org**.
American Diabetes Association titles are also available in bookstores nationwide.